Life Before Birth

Second Edition

The *Humane Fœtus* tho no bigger then a *Green Pea,*
yet is furni∫hed with all its parts.

Antonj van Leeuwenhoek, 1683

Life Before Birth

Second Edition

Marjorie A. England
Senior Lecturer, Pre-Clinical Sciences
Faculty of Medicine
University of Leicester, UK

The Helen Waddell Visiting Professor
School of Biomedical Science
The Queen's University of Belfast, UK

Lately, Honorary Senior Research Fellow
The Royal College of Surgeons of England, UK

Ⓜ Mosby-Wolfe

London Baltimore Barcelona Bogotá Boston Buenos Aires Carlsbad, CA Chicago Madrid Mexico City Milan Naples, FL New York Philadelphia St. Louis Seoul Singapore Sydney Taipei Tokyo Toronto Wiesbaden

Project Managers:	Linda Horrell, Jeremy Theobald
Development Editors:	Simon Pritchard, Lucy Hamilton
Designer:	Marie McNestry
Production:	Siobahn Egan
Index:	Anne McCarthy
Publisher:	Geoff Greenwood

Copyright © 1996 M.A. England

Published in 1996 by Mosby-Wolfe, an imprint of Times Mirror International Publishers Limited

Colour reproduction by Reed Reprographics, Ipswich, Suffolk, UK

Printed by Graphos S.A. Arte sobre papel, Barcelona, Spain

ISBN 0 7234 2474 8 (hbk)

ISBN 0 7234 2475 6 (pbk)

For full details of all Times Mirror International Publishers Limited titles, please write to Times Mirror International Publishers Limited, Lynton House, 7–12 Tavistock Square, London WC1H 9LB, UK.

A CIP catalogue record for this book is available from the British Library.

Library of Congress Cataloging-in-Publication Data applied for.

Contents

Acknowledgements to the Second Edition

In addition to those individuals who kindly allowed me to photograph their collections for the First Edition, the following people and their institutions have generously helped me prepare this second edition.

I am particularly grateful to Dr G. Batcup, Consultant Pathologist, University of Leeds, Dr E.C. Blenkinsopp, Consultant Pathologist, Watford General Hospital, Professor K. Carr and the Anatomy Department of The Queen's University of Belfast (QUB), Professor M. Day, St Thomas' Hospital Medical School (St T), Dr T. El-Sayed, Consultant Radiologist, Watford General Hospital, Dr C. Mills, The Hallam Medical Centre, and Mrs A. Neale, ARDMS, RVT, Southwest Florida Regional Imaging Center, Florida, USA. I am also grateful to The Royal College of Obstetricians and Gynaecologists (RCOG) for access to a collection on permanent loan. I am very grateful for the privilege of using their materials and it is a pleasure to thank them. I am also pleased to thank Professor W. Kilarski, Jagiellonian University, Krakow, Poland, for arranging access to the Anatomical Collection, and Dr J. Karasinski and Dr M. Romek for their assistance. Professor R. Bellairs, University College London, gave assistance and support in the First Edition, but was inadvertently omitted from the acknowledgements.

Dr M. Perry, Senior Lecturer, United Medical and Dental Schools, gave useful advice, as did Mr N. Badham, Lecturer in Clinical Morphology, University of Leicester. Dr J. Wakely, Lecturer, Dr C. Ockleford, Senior Lecturer, and Mr J.N. James, Consultant Oral Surgeon emeritus, University of Leicester, generously gave their time and advice. Dr G. Dickson, Lecturer, The Queen's University of Belfast, kindly advised me on bones and joints. Dr D. Sapunar and Dr K. Vilovic, Medical School, Split, Croatia, advised me on notochord development.

I am also very grateful to Mr J. Bashford, University of Cambridge, who allowed me the rare privilege of consulting Professor J.D. Boyd's notebooks, original data, and specimens prepared by Mr F. Fozzard. Mr B. Logan, Prosector at Cambridge University, and Mrs B. Wells, Librarian, generously gave their time and assistance while I consulted The Boyd Collection at Cambridge University. I am very grateful to the Anatomy Department for allowing me to use this collection recently catalogued with support from The Anatomical Society of Great Britain and Ireland.

Mr M.J. Fenton, St. Thomas' Hospital Medical School, advised me on materials he had prepared and assisted me to photograph them. Mr G. Bryan, The Queen's University of Belfast, also assisted me in photographing materials in his care. Mr S. Rogers, Diagnostic Andrology Clinic, London, gave helpful advice.

I would also like to thank Dr D. Watt, Reader, Charing Cross and Westminster Hospital Medical School, and the Anatomy Department for assistance with material.

I am grateful to Mr D. Adams and Mr I. Indams, University of Leicester, for allowing me to photograph their placental preparation.

Assistance was also received from Mr P. Baines, Watford General Hospital, who generously gave his time. Mr N. Cockcroft, Mrs J. Williams, and Miss D. Meecham, University of Leicester, assisted me in my work. Mr G.L.C. McTurk, Leicester University, gave advice and produced the scanning electron micrographs.

The Leicester University Central Photographic Unit gave assistance and advice. I am grateful to Mr I. Paterson, Mr H. Kowalski, Mr P. Smith, Miss S. Bijl, and Miss U. Sangani for all their help. An especial acknowledgement is made to Mr C. Brookes, whose expert photography enhances this edition, and to Mr K. Garfield's original contributions to the First Edition.

I should like to thank Professor F. Harris, Dean, Faculty of Medicine, for his interest in this book.

I am pleased to thank my publisher Mr G. Greenwood and his team at Mosby-Wolfe for all their advice and support, and in particular, I would like to thank Marie McNestry, for the design work, and my Project Manager, Linda Horrell. Further invaluable assistance on color balance was given by Mr D. Reed of Reed Reprographics.

Finally, I am grateful to Dr J.M. England, Consultant Hematologist, Watford General Hospital, whose encouragement and support have been invaluable.

Acknowledgements

This book has only been possible because of the goodwill and generosity of several people and their institutions. In particular, Professor R.E.M. Bowden, Royal Free Hospital School of Medicine (RFHSM), Professor R.M.H. McMinn, Royal College of Surgeons of England (RCS), Dr R.M. Ransom, Consultant Pathologist, Watford General Hospital, Dr T. El-Sayed, Consultant Radiologist, Watford General Hospital, and Dr G. Slavin, Consultant Pathologist, Northwick Park Hospital, provided access to personal collections of material or ones prepared for their institutions by many workers through several generations. I am very grateful for this privilege.

I am also grateful to Professor T.W.A. Glenister, Charing Cross Hospital Medical School (CCHMS), and to the Anatomy Department for allowing me to photograph some of the specimens in their collection.

I am indebted to Professor I. Craft, Royal Free Hospital, for the photographs of *in vitro* fertilization.

Professor F.R. Johnson, London Hospital School of Medicine (LHSM), allowed me to photograph several specimens from his department.

Professor R.E. Coupland, University of Nottingham, also allowed me to photograph specimens from his departmental collection.

Professor F. Walker, University of Leicester, also gave permission to photograph material.

Dr D. Dooley, lately Her Majesty's Inspector of Anatomy, provided an alizarin red specimen.

Professor H. Nishimura, Professor Emeritus of Anatomy, Kyoto University, kindly provided the photographs of the somite embryos.

I am also grateful for the assistance and advice received from Dr A.J. Palfrey, Charing Cross Hospital Medical School, Dr A. Gulamhusein, University of Leicester, Dr I. Zadawi, Leicester General Hospital, Dr S.A. Ayettey and Dr M.E. Ward, Department of Anatomy, University of Ghana, and Mr R. Watts, Chief Technician, Charing Cross Hospital Medical School, who also allowed me to use his copies of photographs of the radio-opaque studies of fetal circulation. Dr E.C. Blenkinsopp, Consultant Pathologist, Watford General Hospital, Dr A.M.C. Burgess, London Hospital Medical School, Dr J. Wakely, University of Leicester, Dr T. Boulos and Dr C. Tagoe, University of Leicester, Mr G. Bottomley, Chief Technician, University of Leicester, all made specimens available.

Assistance was also received from Miss E. Allen, Hunterian Museum, and Mr B.M. Logan, Department of Anatomy, Royal College of Surgeons of England, Miss M. Hudson, Charing Cross Hospital Medical School, Mr F. Young, Chief Technician, Nottingham University, Mrs S. Barraclough, Watford General Hospital, Mr R.C. Preston, Miss A. Cole, Mr C.G. Brooks, Mr H.J. Kowalski, Mr G.M. Lee, Mr I. Paterson, and Mr G.L.C. McTurk, University of Leicester, and Mr J.E. Cartledge, Leicester General Hospital.

Dr C. Ockleford read the section on the developing fetal membranes and placenta; his constructive advice is gratefully acknowledged. Professor R. Wheeler Haines, Medical College, Baghdad, and Dr J. Wakely, University of Leicester, read the finished text and made suggestions for alterations and clarification. Professor J.L. Emery, University of Sheffield, commented upon the photographs. I am very grateful for their kindness in assuming this task, though I accept full responsibility for any remaining errors or omissions.

I should like to thank Professor F. Beck for his interest and encouragement during the writing of this book.

Dr J.M. England, Consultant Hematologist, Watford General Hospital, kindly assisted and encouraged me throughout the preparation of this book.

I am also grateful to W.B. Saunders Co., Philadelphia, USA, for permission to reproduce the figures provided by Professor H. Nishimura, Kyoto University, which were published in *The Developing Human (Clinically Oriented Embryology)* by Keith L. Moore (1973).

Preface to the Second Edition

In the years following the publication of the First Edition of this book, several laws and social practices have been introduced to closely regulate the use of fetal materials. The result has been a dearth of available specimens, which is largely reflected in these photographs. Wherever possible, new specimens are presented, but there are no new additions in some sections devoted to the older fetal materials. In fact, most of the specimens illustrated in the First Edition are no longer in existence due to the disappearance of some collections.

An attempt has been made to change from Streeter's Horizons to the Carnegie Stages introduced by O'Rahilly and Müller (see Gestational Age). However, the only consistent method of ageing in photographs where the wholemount specimens are no longer available is to rely on the originally reported crown–rump measurement. While this is not ideal, it offers an estimate of age. In some specimens in this book, the ageing given spans two or three Stages to accommodate the crown–rump measurements.

Some, but not all, aspects of normal human development presented are linked by descriptions serving as an *aide-mémoire* of embryology. Only structures of interest and orientation have been labelled for the reader. In some instances, a photograph has been reused to illustrate different features.

It is hoped that this Second Edition will serve the students of medicine and its allied fields to visualize the beauty and three dimensional nature of human embryonic and fetal development.

Preface to the First Edition

This Atlas is intended to illustrate some aspects of normal human development *in utero*. The descriptions accompanying the photographs serve as a link between them and as an *aide memoire* of embryology. The reader would be well advised also to consult the textbooks listed in Suggestions for Further Reading.

All the illustrations contained in this book are from human specimens, many of which were prepared over 40 years ago. A number of specimens had previously been mis-sexed; it is hoped the illustrations in this book will help prevent such confusion in the future. It must also be remembered that, although embryos of identical lengths are comparable, each organ is individual in its rate of growth and differentiation. For example, the arm primordia in one embryo of 12 mm crown–rump length may be present only as buds whilst in another they may already have differentiated into arm, forearm and hand sections.

Some of the specimens appear poorly dissected, but when compared with the head of a pin (p. 125)* the difficulties with dissection become apparent. Many of the smallest specimens were dissected with cactus spines mounted on handles as conventional instruments were too large. Some early specimens have crystals of fixative on their surface which were impossible to remove without damaging the specimen.

It was not intended to label every structure present on a specimen, but rather to label structures of interest and orientation for the reader. Photographs illustrating several points may be used on more than one occasion.

It is hoped this book will assist students of medicine, nursing, and the allied fields to visualize the structures which hereto have been largely illustrated by line drawings.

*In the Second Edition this is p. 127.

Terminology

1a. Terminology used to indicate top, bottom, front and back.

1b. Terminology used to indicate movement toward and away from the midline.

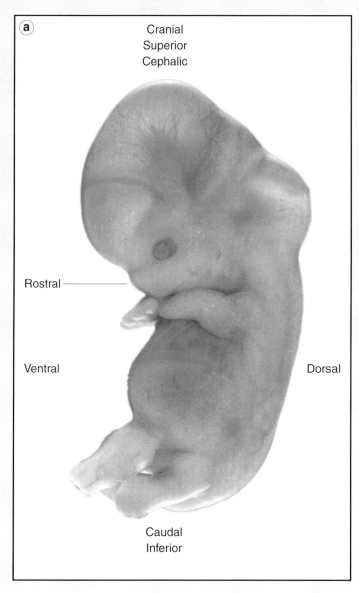

ROSTRAL: A structure's relationship to the nose.

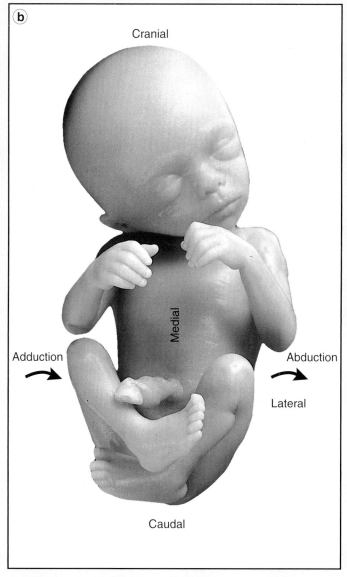

ADDUCTION: Movement toward the midline.
ABDUCTION: Movement away from the midline.

Planes of Section

2. An embryo or fetus is usually sectioned in the following planes:

Coronal (frontal)

Horizontal (transverse)

Sagittal
(median or longitudinal)

The arrows indicate the direction of the plane of section.

● Early embryos are flexed and it is possible in one transverse section to cross both the head and heart regions.

Gestational Age

An estimate of gestational age can be made by measuring the embryo or fetus. Various methods of measurement have been developed each with its own limitations and inaccuracies. Crown–rump and crown–heel lengths are the commonest measurements; this book uses crown–rump (CR) length in mm. Crown–heel (CH) lengths are difficult to measure because the legs are often flexed in different positions. Foot-length measurements are also used as a guide to developmental age.

Most methods based on measurements are inaccurate because the specimens can be changed by stretching in handling or shrinking in fixation.

A series of developing external and internal features of an embryo is a more accurate measure of maturity. Streeter (1942, 1948) presented a series of Horizons I–XXIII which he used to age embryos until Day 47. These descriptions were based on a *true age*, stretching from fertilization at Time 0 to term at Week 38 (Day 266). Recent research has necessitated some slight alterations of Streeter's original tables. This book uses O'Rahilly and Müller's Carnegie Stages (O'Rahilly and Müller, 1987), which have replaced Streeter's Horizons. The reader is also advised to consult Iffy *et al.* (1967), O'Rahilly (1973), and Gasser (1975).

Most clinicians do not know the fertilization date; the only date available to them from the mother is the first day of the last menstrual period. They use this date to assign a *menstrual age*, stretching from Time 0, which is usually 14 days before fertilization, to term at Week 40 (9.2 calendar months).

In this book, descriptions of early development are based on the fertilization date and expressed as true ages in hours, days, or weeks and as Carnegie Stages. For the very late fetuses the dates are often based on the last menstrual period and expressed as menstrual ages in calendar months. Readers should be aware that other workers have used lunar months (4 weeks) rather than calendar months; term is 10 lunar months from the first day of the last menstrual period

REFERENCES

Gasser, R. (1975) *Atlas of Human Embryos*. Hagerstown, Harper & Row.

Iffy, L., Shepard, T.H., Jakobovits, A., Lemire, R.J. and Kerner, P. (1967) *Acta Anat.*, **66**, 178–186.

O'Rahilly, R. (1973) Carnegie Institution of Washington Publication 631.

O'Rahilly, R. and Müller, F. (1987) Carnegie Institution of Washington Publication 637.

Streeter, G.L. (1942) Carnegie Institution of Washington Publications, **30**, 211–245.

Streeter, G.L. (1948) Carnegie Institution of Washington Publications, **32**, 133–203.

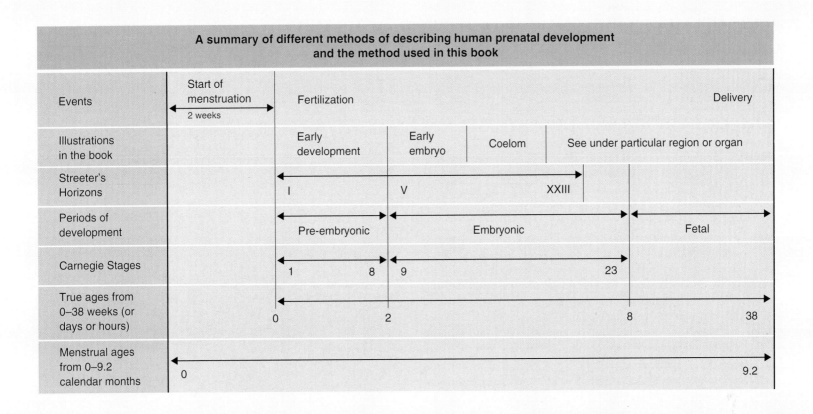

A summary of different methods of describing human prenatal development and the method used in this book

Events	Start of menstruation 2 weeks	Fertilization			Delivery
Illustrations in the book		Early development	Early embryo	Coelom	See under particular region or organ
Streeter's Horizons		I	V	XXIII	
Periods of development		Pre-embryonic	Embryonic		Fetal
Carnegie Stages		1 8	9 23		
True ages from 0–38 weeks (or days or hours)		0 2		8	38
Menstrual ages from 0–9.2 calendar months	0				9.2

CROWN–RUMP

3a. Crown–rump (CR) measurement from the crown of the head to the rump of the embryo or fetus.

CROWN–HEEL

3b. Crown–heel (CH) measurement from the crown of the head to the heel of the fetus. (Standing height.)

Normal Series of Development

The pre-embryonic period

Stages 1–2 Fertilization to the third day. These stages include the single cell fertilized (penetrated) oocyte and segmentation (cleavage) of the oocyte (ootid) to form the zygote composed of 12–16 cells (morula). Approximately 0.1–0.2 mm in diameter. Week 1.

Stage 3 Day 4. The free (unattached) blastocyst stage. Approximately 32 cells up to 200 cells 0.1–0.2 mm in diameter. Stages 1–3 are referred to as pre-implantation stages.

Stage 4 Days 5–6. The blastocyst attaches to the endometrium and the beginning of implantation. Approximately 0.1–0.2 mm in diameter.

Stage 5 Days 7–12. The implanted embryo is embedded more deeply in the uterine endometrium. The amniotic and exocoelomic cavities are present. This stage may be referred to as the previllous stage because there are no definite chorionic villi. This stage is usually subdivided on the basis of trophoblastic development. The extraembryonic mesoblast forms. Approximately 0.1–0.2 mm in diameter. Week 2.

Stages 6–8 Days 13–18. These stages may be referred to as presomitic. The chorionic villi branch, the primitive streak and notochordal process appear, as well as the notochordal and neurenteric canals. Toward the end of the period, the neural plate and groove appear and the neural folds may be present. Approximately 0.2 mm CR in Stage 6 to approximately 1.0–1.5 mm CR in Stage 8. Weeks 2–3.

- Normal males usually produce more than 100 million sperm per ml of semen.
- Semen containing less than 20 million sperm per ml is likely to be infertile.

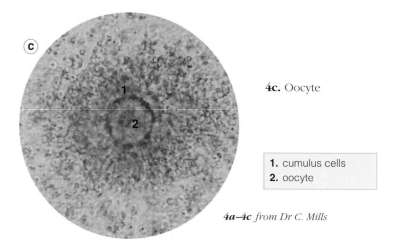

4c. Oocyte

| 1. cumulus cells |
| 2. oocyte |

4a–4c from Dr C. Mills

4d. Stage 1. The immature oocyte with one polar body after maturation *in vitro* for 48 h.

| 1. oocyte |
| 2. polar body |
| 3. zona pellucida |

4d from Professor I. Craft

4a. Sperm, viewed by phase microscopy.

4b. Sperm stained with fluorescent pisum sativum lectin for the acrosomal contents.

| 1. head |
| 2. reacted acrosome |
| 3. sperm |
| 4. tail |
| 5. unreacted (or intact) acrosome |

4e and **4f.** Stage 2. The oocyte divides by mitosis and the resulting new embryonic cells are smaller in size.

4e. Two-cell zygote.

4f. Four-cell zygote.

| 1. cumulus cells |
| 2. embryonic cells |
| 3. sperm |
| 4. vitelline membrane |

4g–4i. Stage 2. Embryos matured *in vitro.*

4g. Eight-cell zygote.

> **1.** cell (blastomere)
> **2.** corona radiata
> **3.** zona pellucida

4b *from Professor I. Craft*
4g *and* **4i** *from Dr C. Mills*

4h. Nine-cell zygote after maturation *in vitro* for 72 h.

4i. Zygote.

The embryonic period

Stages 9–10 Days 20–22. Stages 9–13 may be referred to as the somitic stages. The first somites (1–12) appear, and the neural folds begin to fuse. The head and tail folds are apparent. Two pharyngeal arch bars are present, the two heart tubes are fused in the midline, and contractions begin. Approximately 1.5–2.5 mm CR in Stage 9 to 1.5–3 mm CR in Stage 10. Weeks 3–4.

Stages 11–12 Days 24–26. The optic vesicle and otocyst are present. The rostral and caudal neuropores close and the forebrain and hindbrain and their rhombomeres are distinguished easily. The brain bends at the midbrain flexure. The primordia of the lungs, liver, stomach, pancreas, thyroid gland, and mesonephric tubules are evident. The upper limb buds appear, and 3–4 pharyngeal bars are present. There are 13–29 somites and the embryo is approximately 2.5–4.5 mm CR in Stage 11 to 3–5 mm CR in Stage 12. Week 4.

5a–5c *from Professor H. Nishimura*

> **1.** anterior (rostral) neuropore
> **2.** brain
> **3.** caudal
> **4.** cephalic
> **5.** neural tube
> **6.** posterior (caudal) neuropore
> **7.** somites

5a. Stage 10 (Day 22 ± 1 day). The cephalic and caudal ends of the embryo can be distinguished at this stage, as well as right and left sides.

5b. Stage 10 (Day 22 ± 1 day). The neural tube is fusing opposite the somites. The anterior and posterior neuropores remain widely opened.

5c. Stage 11 (Day 24 ± 1 day). The anterior neuropore is closing while the posterior neuropore remains open.

Stage 13 Day 28. There are approximately 30+ somites at this stage. The leg bud appears, so all four limb buds are visible. The heart bulges from the body. The otic vesicle is now closed and the lens disc forms. The blood circulation is now well established. Approximately 4–6 mm CR. Week 4.

Stage 14 Day 32. The secondary brain vesicles begin to form and the spinal nerves sprout. The optic cup begins to develop. In the heart, the semilunar valves begin to form as do the coronary vessels. In the urogenital system, the metanephric kidneys begin to develop. Approximately 5–7 mm CR. Week 5.

Stage 15 Day 33. The axons of the primary olfactory neurons reach the telencephalon. The lens vesicle is present, and the medial and lateral nasal processes form. The cranial nerve motor nuclei, sensory and parasympathetic cranial nerve ganglia begin to form. The genital tubercle is present as is the hand plate. Approximately 7–9 mm CR.

Stage 16 Day 37. The foot plate appears on the lower limb bud. Pigment appears in the retina of the eye and the auricular hillocks of the external ear are apparent. The lumen of the gut proliferates. In the urogenital system, the genital ridges appear. Approximately 8–11 mm CR. Week 6.

6. Stage 12 (Day 26 ± 1 day). The arm bud is just appearing. 3.5 mm CR

1. branchial arch
2. embryonic membranes
3. forebrain prominence
4. heart bulge
5. tail

6 from Dr E.C. Blenkinsopp

7. Stage 13 (Day 28). The embryo is flexed in a 'C' shape. The head, tail, and arm bud are distinguished easily. Branchial arches are present and the heart bulges prominently.

1. arm
2. branchial arches
3. head
4. heart bulge
5. somites
6. tail
7. umbilical stalk

7 from Professor H. Nishimura

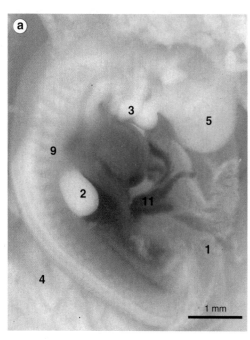

8a. Stage 13 (Day 28). The arm bud is present. 4–6 mm CR

8b from CCHMS

8b. Stage 14 (Day 32). The leg bud is present. 6 mm CR

1. amnion
2. arm bud
3. branchial arches
4. chorion
5. head
6. heart bulge
7. leg bud
8. lens invagination
9. somites
10. tail
11. umbilical cord

Stage 17 Day 41. Finger rays are apparent. In the lungs, the divisions of the bronchopulmonary segments are appearing. In the head, the cerebellar plate is present, as are the dental laminae and nasolacrimal groove. The subcardinal vein system begins to form. Approximately 11–14 mm CR.

9a. Stage 17 (Day 41). The hand plates have developed and the digital rays are present. 12 mm CR

9b. Stage 17 (Day 41). The embryo *in situ* in the uterus. 12.6 mm CR

1. arm bud (with hand plate and digital ridges)
2. branchial arches
3. chorion
4. embryo
5. embryonic membrane
6. eye
7. forebrain
8. heart bulge
9. hindbrain
10. leg bud
11. liver bulge
12. somites
13. tail
14. umbilical cord
15. uterus

9c. Stages 17–18 (Days 41–44). The diamond-shaped hindbrain is clearly visible and the arm bud has an elbow. 14 mm CR

9b *and* **9c** *from RCS*

Stages 18–19   Days 44–48. The trunk begins to elongate and the body assumes a more cuboidal shape. The elbow region appears and the toe rays are apparent. Ossification may begin. On the head, the eyelid folds begin to form and the tip of the nose is distinct. Approximately 13–17 mm CR in Stage 18 and 17–20 mm CR in Stage 19. Week 7.

• Using ultrasound, the first movements are apparent.

Stage 20   Days 50–51. The upper limbs begin to bend at the elbows and the fingers curve slightly over the cardiac region. The lens cavity is obliterated and a suture begins to form. The cerebral hemispheres cover two-thirds of the diencephalon. Approximately 21–23 mm CR. Week 8.

Stages 21–23   Days 52–57. The hands and feet approach each other in the midline and the limbs have increased in length. The forearm ascends to a level above the shoulder. The head is becoming erect. The eyes are largely open, but the eyelids may be beginning to fuse medially and laterally. The rhombencephalon is highly organized. The gut tube recanalizes. The external genitalia are well developed. Approximately 22–32 mm CR.

1. arm
2. ear
3. elbow
4. eye
5. forebrain
6. heart bulge
7. hindbrain
8. liver bulge
9. midbrain
10. midgut herniation
11. mouth
12. notched hand plate
13. umbilical cord

10a. Stage 19 (Days 47–48). The arms curve over the heart bulge and the toe rays are present on the foot. 20 mm CR

1. arm
2. ear
3. elbow
4. eye
5. foot
6. forebrain bulge
7. hand
8. knee
9. liver bulge
10. midbrain bulge
11. mouth
12. nose
13. ribs
14. tail
15. toes
16. umbilical cord

10b. Stage 22 (Day 54). The toes have formed and the feet approach the midline. 25 mm CR

10c. Stage 22 (Day 54). 27 mm CR

10d. Stage 23 (Days 56–57). 28 mm CR

The fetal period

Week 8 At the end of Week 8 the embryonic period is complete and the fetal period begins. This period is characterized by the rapid growth of the fetus (especially between Weeks 9–20) and the further differentiation of the organs and tissues formed in the embryonic period.

Weeks 9–12 The head at Week 9 is almost half of the fetus. With the rapid growth, the body length (CR) doubles by Week 12, but the head grows more slowly. The neck lengthens and extends so the chin no longer contacts the body.

The eyelids meet, fuse, and the eyes remain closed until Week 25. Fingernails appear on the digits. The upper limb becomes disproportionately large.

The midgut, which was herniated into the umbilical cord, returns to the enlarged abdominal cavity (Week 10). Bile is secreted.

Distinguishing features of the external genitalia appear in Week 9, and fully differentiate into male (♂) or female (♀) by Week 12.

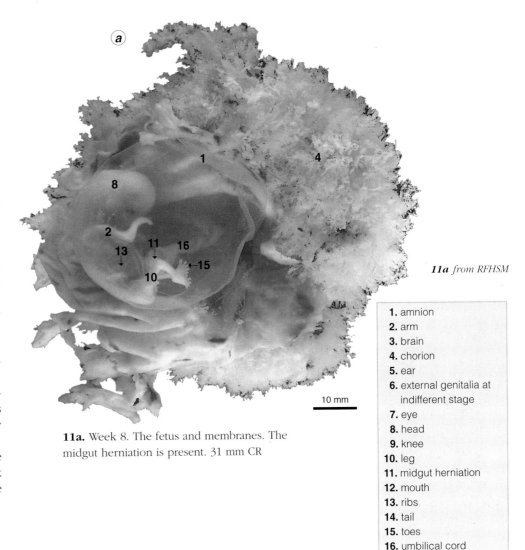

11a from RFHSM

10 mm

11a. Week 8. The fetus and membranes. The midgut herniation is present. 31 mm CR

1. amnion
2. arm
3. brain
4. chorion
5. ear
6. external genitalia at indifferent stage
7. eye
8. head
9. knee
10. leg
11. midgut herniation
12. mouth
13. ribs
14. tail
15. toes
16. umbilical cord

5 mm

5 mm

5 mm

5 mm

11b. Week 8. The external genitalia are beginning to differentiate. 39 mm CR

11c. Week 9. The head is almost half the fetal length. As the head extends and the chin is raised from the thorax the neck develops. The eyelids have fused. 44 mm CR

11d. Week 9. The fingernails appear about this time. 46 mm CR

11e. Week 10. The fetus has doubled in length since Week 7 and the midgut herniation returns to the enlarged abdomen. 60 mm CR ♂

1. arm
2. ear
3. eye
4. foot
5. placenta
6. umbilical cord

12a from RCOG

12a. Week 12. The ear has moved from the neck on to the head. The eyes have moved to the front of the face. 85 mm CR ♀

12b. Week 12. The fetus and membranes. 85 mm CR ♂

10 mm

1. ear
2. eye
3. umbilical cord

13a. Week 13. The skin is very thin and the blood vessels are easily distinguished. 92 mm CR ♀

13b. Week 13. The fetus may suck its thumb from this stage. 97 mm CR ♂

13c. Week 13. 98 mm CR ♀

13c from RFSHM

1. ear
2. eye
3. umbilical cord

13d. Week 14. 105 mm CR ♀

13e. Week 14. The nails are well formed. 106 mm CR ♀

13f. Week 14. The lower limb is longer than the upper limb at this stage of development. Note the umbilical cord looped around the neck. 106 mm CR ♂

13g. Week 14. Fine lanugo hairs are present on the head. The attachment of the umbilical cord is low on the abdomen. 110 mm CR ♂

Weeks 13–16 Rapid growth continues. On the erect head the eyes have moved onto the front of the face, but are still widely separated. The external ear is differentiating and has moved onto the side of the head from the upper neck.

Ossification is progressing rapidly. The skeleton is clearly outlined on radiographs of the fetus. Lanugo hairs cover the body.

13f from RFHSM

13g from Dr G. Batcup

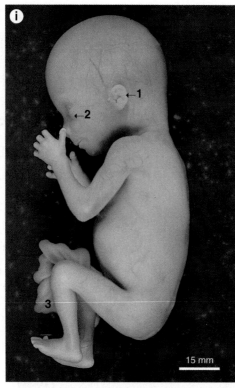

1. ear
2. eye
3. umbilical cord

13h. Week 14. 120 mm CR ♂

13i. Week 14. Limb movements become coordinated. 120 mm CR ♂

14a. Week 15. Brown fat begins to form in this month. 130 mm CR ♀

14b. Week 16. 140 mm CR ♂

14c. Week 16. 140 mm CR ♀

14b from RCOG

15e from RCOG

Weeks 17–20 The rapid growth rate slows down. The final relative proportions of the parts of the lower limb are reached. Sebaceous glands become active and *vernix caseosa* forms to cover and protect the skin from the macerating amniotic fluid.

Myelination of the spinal cord begins.

Brown fat forms. The mother becomes conscious of fetal movements (quickening).

1. ear
2. eye
3. foot
4. mouth
5. umbilical cord

15a. Week 17. Parts of the leg reach their relative proportions in this month. 141 mm CR ♀

15b. Week 17. Fetal movements are present which the mother can consciously feel in the abdomen. 144 mm CR ♀

15c. Week 18. 152 mm CR ♂

15d. Week 18. The sebaceous glands become active and *vernix caseosa* forms to protect the skin from the amniotic fluid. 152 mm CR ♂

15e. Week 18. 160 mm CR ♂

(f)

15f. Week 18. The fetus *in utero.* 160 mm CR ♂

15g. Week 20. The eyelids and eyebrows are very well developed as are the fingernails. 185 mm CR ♀

15g from RCOG

1. abdomen
2. ear
3. eye
4. foot
5. hand
6. knee
7. umbilical cord
8. uterus

16a. Week 21. 200 mm CR ♂

16a from CCHMS

Weeks 21–25 The eyelids and eyebrows are well developed. The lanugo darkens and there is more *vernix caseosa*. The skin may be very wrinkled due to the lack of subcutaneous fat and a relative increase in the growth of the skin. Fingernails are present.

The face and body generally assume the appearance of the infant at birth. Fetuses born from Week 25 onwards are usually viable.

10 mm

16b from CCHMS

16b. Week 22. Gravid uterus with fetus *in situ*. Posterior wall of uterus has been removed.

17a–17j. Normal series of development to show the relative sizes of the growing embryo and fetus. **a.** Stage 19, 18 mm CR. **b.** Week 8, 33 mm CR. **c.** Week 9, 44 mm CR. **d.** Week 10, 60 mm CR ♂. **e.** Week 13, 90 mm CR ♂. **f.** Week 14, 110 mm CR ♂. **g.** Week 17, 150 mm CR ♂. **h.** Week 18, 160 mm CR ♀. **i.** Week 19, 180 mm CR ♂. **j.** Week 23, 225 mm CR ♀.

a 10 mm	b 10 mm	c 10 mm	d 10 mm	e 10 mm	f 10 mm	g 10 mm
Stage 19	Week 8	Week 9	Week 10	Week 13	Week 14	Week 17

17e–17j from RCOG

(h) 10 mm

(i) 10 mm

(j) 10 mm

Week 18

Week 19

Week 23

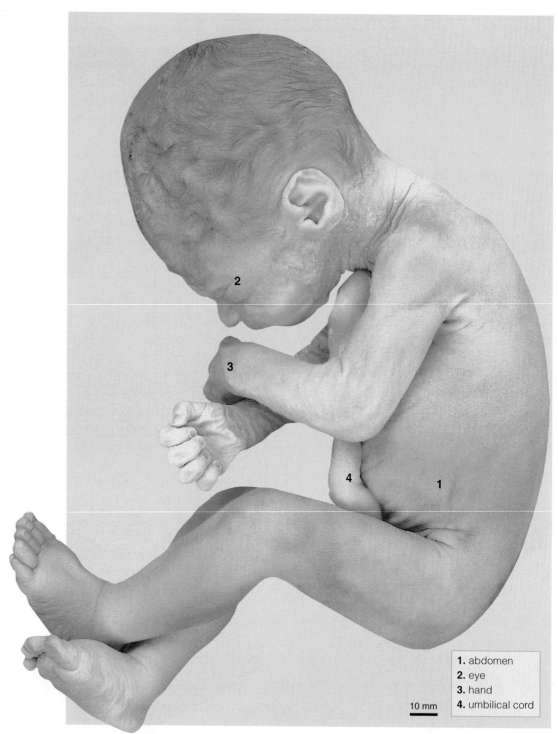

1. abdomen
2. eye
3. hand
4. umbilical cord

10 mm

18. Week 24. 228 mm CR ♂

19a. Week 26. A section of the anterior wall of the uterus to show the attachment of the fetus to the placenta. 250 mm CR

19b. Week 28. The fetus *in situ* with a 'true' knot in the umbilical cord. The testes are descending into the scrotum.

20 mm

19a from CCHMS

1. abdomen
2. eye
3. hand
4. maternal ovary
5. placenta
6. umbilical cord
7. umbilical cord with knot
8. uterus

20 mm

19b from CCHMS

Weeks 26–29 The eyes are open again and the eyebrows and eyelashes are well developed. The pupillary membrane disappears. The scalp hairs are becoming long and the body generally becomes plump and round as subcutaneous fat is deposited.

Weeks 30–34 The body is becoming plumper and the skin is pink. Toenails are present and the testes are descending. The fingernails have reached the tips of the fingers.

Weeks 35–38 The body is plump. The toenails have reached the tips of the toes. Almost all the lanugo hairs have been shed and the skin is covered with *vernix caseosa*. The umbilicus is central in the abdomen. The testes have descended into the scrotum, but the ovaries are still above the level of the pelvic brim and do not reach their final position by birth. Brain myelination begins.

During the final weeks, approximately 14 g of fat a day is laid down. The neonate weighs about 3400 g and is about 360 mm CR.

The male infant normally weighs more than the female infant at birth.

- Clinicians divide pregnancy into three parts, or trimesters (each three calendar months). Natural abortions usually occur during the first trimester.
- Prematurely born male infants may have undescended testes.

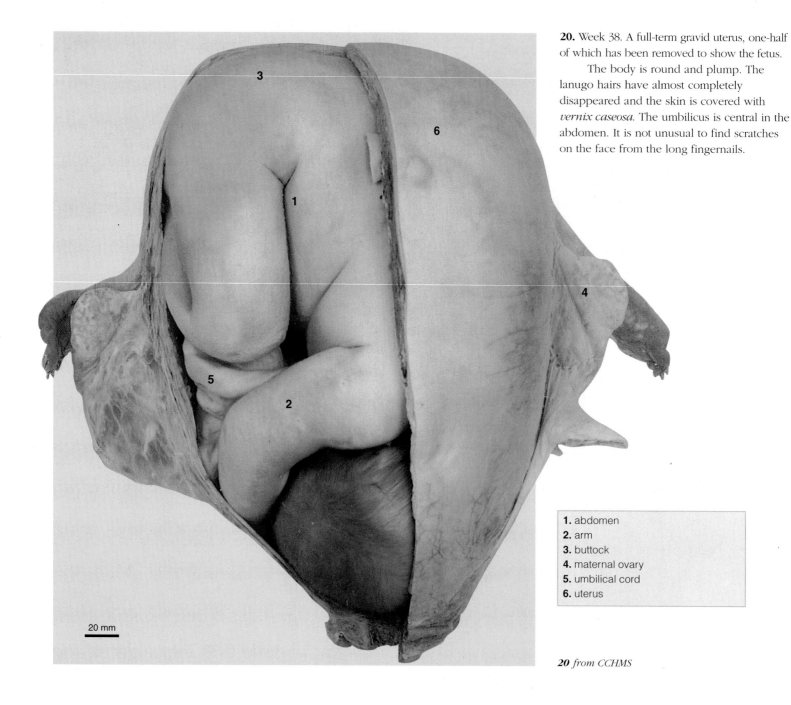

20 mm

20. Week 38. A full-term gravid uterus, one-half of which has been removed to show the fetus.

The body is round and plump. The lanugo hairs have almost completely disappeared and the skin is covered with *vernix caseosa*. The umbilicus is central in the abdomen. It is not unusual to find scratches on the face from the long fingernails.

| **1.** abdomen |
| **2.** arm |
| **3.** buttock |
| **4.** maternal ovary |
| **5.** umbilical cord |
| **6.** uterus |

20 from CCHMS

Ultrasound

Development *in utero* is assessed very accurately by using ultrasound methods to scan the maternal abdomen. Gestational age can be estimated at different periods in development by using the chorionic (gestational) sac volume, crown–rump (CR) length, biparietal diameter, femur length, head and abdominal circumferences, and cerebellum. The most accurate measurements are the biparietal diameter and the femur length in the second trimester.

The membranes are detectable by transabdominal scanning at Week 6 and the embryo from Week 7. The embryo or fetus can be measured and its viability confirmed by heart movements. Multiple conceptions can be recognized in the first trimester, and the placental positions in the second trimester.

During the first trimester, the CR length is measured giving an estimate of age which is accurate to within 4 days. From Week 12 flexion makes the CR measurement more unreliable. The biparietal diameter of the head, which is ossifying between Weeks 11 and 12, is used instead. The date of delivery can be predicted to within 7 days if the biparietal diameter is measured prior to Week 24. Later in pregnancy (Weeks 34–38) the biparietal measurement becomes inaccurate.

From Week 12 to term, the femur length is a very reliable indicator of normal growth. The majority of women are initially scanned at Weeks 18–20 and subsequently scanned again if this is clinically indicated. The timing of the second scan is dependent upon the clinical problem.

In transvaginal ultrasonography, the probe is placed within the vagina and is closely related to the embryo. This method allows the clinician to obtain a very accurate assessment of a problem arising within the first trimester, i.e., in a suspected ectopic pregnancy, blighted ovum, threatened abortion.

In implantation after *in vitro* fertilization studies, the CR length has been determined as early as 25 days. The chorionic (gestational) sac median diameter can also be measured; e.g., a 2–3 mm median sac diameter is about Day 16–17. Even heart movements and umbilical blood flow can be assessed accurately using color flow Doppler imaging.

21a. Scan of the placenta of a Week 16 fetus to determine the placental site in relation to the maternal uterine os.

1. maternal abdomen
2. maternal uterine os
3. placenta

21b. Scan of a Week 16 fetus with a normal cerebellum.

21a–30d from Dr T. El-Sayed

1. cerebellum
2. falx cerebri
3. lateral ventricles

Several developmental abnormalities can be detected by ultrasound, e.g., spine abnormalities, limb defects, organ anomalies, etc. X-rays are a very accurate method of assessment, but they are only rarely used now because of the effects of radiation on the developing fetus, e.g., leukemia later in life.

- Embryonic heart pulsations may be detected by ultrasound methods as early as Week 6 of gestation.
- Fetal sex can be identified from Week 14 and could be important in sex-linked conditions.
- Fetal kidneys can be identified at Week 14 and from Week 16 the normal bladder will empty every 40–45 minutes.
- The blood supply to the fetus via the umbilical vessels can be assessed using a transvaginal probe with color flow Doppler.

21c. Scan of a Week 16 fetus illustrating the abdominal circumference.

1. abdominal circumference
2. maternal abdominal surface
3. maternal bladder
4. stomach (fetal)

21d. Scan of a Week 16+ fetus. The relative proportions of the leg are assessed during this period.

1. femur
2. fibula
3. foot
4. knee
5. thigh
6. tibia

22a. Scan of a Week 17 fetal face.

1. lens of eye
2. mouth
3. nose

22b. Scan of the profile of a Week 17 fetal face and thorax.

1. eye
2. mouth
3. neck
4. nose
5. ribs

22c. Scan of a Week 17 fetus to illustrate the spinal column.

1. ear
2. face
3. fetal head
4. maternal abdominal surface
5. occiput of head
6. vertebrae of spinal column

22d. Scan of a Week 17 head and upper limb.

1. amniotic cavity
2. head
3. humerus
4. maternal abdominal surface
5. metacarpals
6. phalanges
7. radius
8. ulna

22e. Scan of a Week 17 hand.

1. index finger
2. maternal abdominal surface
3. metacarpals
4. phalanges
5. thumb

22f. Scan of a Week 17 thorax and abdomen.

1. arm
2. diaphragm
3. heart
4. liver
5. lung
6. maternal abdominal surface

23. Scan of the profile of a Week 22+ fetus.

1. arm
2. auricle of ear
3. eye
4. frontal bone
5. mouth
6. nose
7. occiput of head
8. shoulder

24a. Scan of a Week 18+ fetus to illustrate the chambers of the heart.

1. atrium
2. lower limb
3. maternal abdominal surface
4. ventricle

24b. Scan of a Week 18 fetus. Coronal view of the kidneys and bladder.

1. bladder
2. buttocks
3. innominate bone
4. kidneys
5. maternal abdominal surface
6. ribs
7. spinal column

25. Scan of a Week 26 fetal foot.

1. maternal abdominal surface
2. plantar surface
3. toes

26. Scan of a Week 29 fetus to assess the length of the femur.

1. femur length
2. maternal abdominal surface

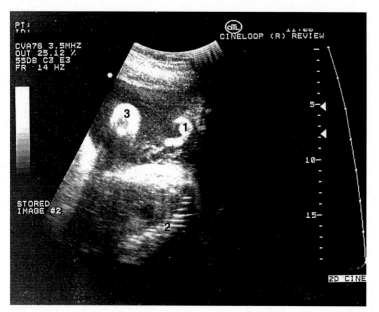

27. Scan of the auricle of the ear of a Week 32 fetus.

1. auricle of ear
2. ribs
3. shoulder

28. Scan of a Week 33 fetus.

1. fetal abdomen
2. kidneys
3. maternal abdominal surface
4. vertebra

29a and **29b.** Scan of a Week 20 fetus to measure the biparietal diameter and head circumference of the skull.

1. biparietal diameter
2. head circumference
3. maternal abdominal surface

TWINS

30a. Scan of twins

1. circumference of abdomen
2. fetal abdomen
3. maternal abdominal surface

30b. Scan of the measurement of one limb of the first twin.

1. gestational sac
2. limb measurement
3. maternal abdominal surface

30c. Scan of the first twin's gestational sac.

| 1. gestational sac |
| 2. maternal abdominal surface |

30d. Scan of the measurement of one limb of the second twin.

| 1. limb measurement |
| 2. maternal abdominal surface |

COLOR FLOW DOPPLER

31a. Cine scan to illustrate fetal viability.

31a–31b from Mrs A. Neale

| 1. fetus |
| 2. gestational sac |

31b. Still of scan to measure CR length.

| 1. CR measurement |
| 2. gestational sac |

31c. Scan of blood flow through the pulsating heart.

1. heart
2. red (cardiac chamber)
3. blue (cardiac chamber)

31d and **31e.** Scan to illustrate blood flow through the umbilical cord.

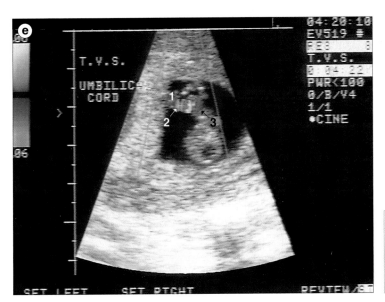

1. umbilical cord
2. oxygenated blood
   (vein: red)
3. deoxygenated blood
   (artery: blue)

31f and **31g.** Scan of blood flow through the chorionic plate.

1. chorionic plate

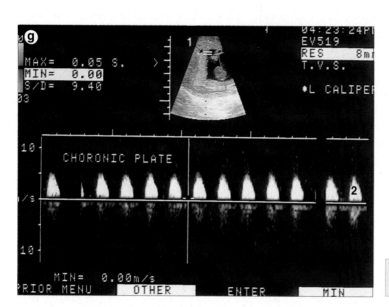

1. cursor sample
2. pulsations

31h. Scan to assess the amniotic contents in amniocentesis.

1. amnion
2. gestational sac

Early Development

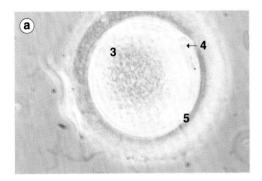

32a. Stage 1. The immature oocyte with one polar body after maturation *in vitro* for 48 h.

32a and *32b* *from Professor I. Craft*

32b. Stage 2. The nine-cell zygote after maturation *in vitro* for 72 h.

1. cell (blastomere)	**4.** polar body
2. corona radiata	**5.** zona pellucida
3. oocyte	

Development of the embryo begins at Stage 1 when a sperm fertilizes an oocyte and together they form a zygote. As the zygote travels down the uterine (Fallopian) tube it divides (cleavage) into two blastomeres at about 30 h after fertilization. The cells continue to divide until a ball or morula of 12 or more cells is present. The morula enters the uterus, and at Day 4 fluid from the uterine cavity enters the morula and the cells rearrange themselves to form the blastocyst. Some of the cells form a single-layered hollow ball called the trophoblast which will form part of the placenta. Other cells form the inner cell mass embryoblast attached to one pole of the trophoblast. The blastocyst is enclosed in an acellular layer, the zona pellucida.

The blastocyst lies free in the uterine cavity for about 2 days, then loses its zona pellucida at Days 4–5, and attaches to the maternal endometrium by Days 5–6. The trophoblast cells invade the endometrium and gradually differentiate into two layers; cytotrophoblast and syncytiotrophoblast (outermost layer).

As the embryo differentiates, endoderm (hypoblast) forms at about Day 7 from cells of the inner cell mass which are closest to the blastocyst cavity. Small spaces appear in the remaining inner cell mass which coalesce to form the amniotic cavity (see Amnion).

The remaining cells of the inner cell mass form the ectoderm and mesoderm layers during Week 3. The embryo is then a bilaminar embryonic disc, with the amnion above and the blastocyst cavity below. Hypoblast cells migrate and form an inner exocoelomic lining (Heuser's membrane) to the blastocyst, so enclosing the exocoelomic cavity (primary yolk sac). Further hypoblast cells delaminate to form extraembryonic mesoderm around the amnion and yolk sac. The extraembryonic mesoderm increases and spaces appear in it, which coalesce to form the extraembryonic coelom. This coelom surrounds the amnion and yolk stalk, except at the connecting (body or umbilical) stalk. As the extraembryonic coelom develops, the secondary yolk sac forms below the embryonic endoderm. The extraembryonic mesoderm is also split into two layers; somatic (somatopleuric) mesoderm lining the trophoblast and amnion and splanchnic (splanchnopleuric) mesoderm lining the yolk sac.

Together the extraembryonic somatic mesoderm and trophoblast form the chorion, while the cavity is the extraembryonic coelom (chorionic cavity).

Early Embryo

The embryo is a bilaminar disc with a localized thickening of the endoderm, called the prochordal plate, at the future site of the mouth. The embryo at Day 15 has reached the primitive streak stage, the streak having a primitive knot or node at its cephalic end with a primitive pit. Recent studies have reported the primitive streak appearing by Days 12–14. The primitive streak gives the first indication of the cephalic, caudal, dorsal, ventral, right and left sides of the embryo.

By Day 16 ectoderm cells which have migrated toward the primitive streak invaginate to form intraembryonic mesoderm cells. Some of these cells cranial to the knot form the notochordal process, while other mesoderm cells migrate between the ectoderm and endoderm layers until they reach the margins of the disc and become continuous with the amniotic and yolk sac mesoderm. Some of these cells form the cardiogenic area. By the middle of Week 3 mesoderm cells are present throughout the embryo except in the regions of the oropharyngeal membrane (prochordal plate), cloacal membrane, and notochordal process. Mesoderm cells are produced actively until the end of Week 4. The primitive streak becomes relatively diminished in size as the notochord increases in length. The primitive pit extends into the notochordal process to form the notochordal canal. The notochordal process fuses with the underlying endoderm layer and where fusion occurs degeneration takes place and the notochordal canal becomes continuous with the yolk sac. The roof or notochordal plate upfolds to form the notochord itself and the endoderm again forms a continuous layer ventral to the notochord. For a short period the amniotic cavity and yolk sac (umbilical vesicle) are continuous through the neurenteric canal, which is completely obliterated as the notochord forms fully.

While the notochord is developing, the overlying ectoderm forms neuroectoderm which will give rise to the central nervous system. The neuroectoderm has a neural groove and neural folds which fuse by the end of Week 3 and form the neural tube. The neural crest cells form from some of the more lateral neuroectoderm cells which are not incorporated into the neural tube.

1. amniotic cavity
2. cytotrophoblast
3. ectoderm
4. endoderm
5. endometrium
6. exocoelomic membrane
7. extra-embryonic endoderm
8. lacunae
9. primary yolk sac
10. secondary yolk sac
11. trophoblast
12. uterine glands

33a. Stage 5 (Days 7–12). The early blastocyst embryo sectioned transversely. The endometrial epithelium has regenerated over the implanted ovum.

33b. A higher magnification of the embryo in **33a** in a slightly more posterior transverse section.

33c. Stage 6 (Day 13). The bilaminar embryo sectioned transversely.

33a–33c from CCHMS

33d. Stage 7 (Day 16). The secondary yolk sac is present. The allantois first appears during this stage.

33d from QUB

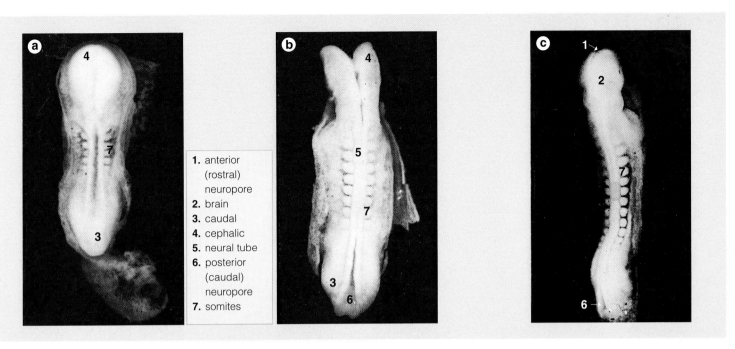

34a. Stage 10 (Day 22 ± 1 day). The cephalic and caudal ends of the embryo can be distinguished at this stage, as well as right and left sides.

34b. Stage 10 (Day 22 ± 1 day). The neural tube is fusing opposite the somites. The anterior and posterior neuropores remain widely opened.

34c. Stage 11 (Day 24 ± 1 day). The anterior neuropore is closing while the posterior neuropore remains open.
34a–34c from Professor H. Nishimura

1. anterior (rostral) neuropore
2. brain
3. caudal
4. cephalic
5. neural tube
6. posterior (caudal) neuropore
7. somites

35a and **35b.** Stage 6 (Day 14). A sagittal section of a gravid uterus.

1. cervix
2. decidua basalis
3. decidua capsularis
4. decidua parietalis
5. uterine cavity
6. uterus

10 mm

35a and 35b from RFHSM

2 mm

As the notochord and neural tube form, the mesoderm adjacent to the midline forms paraxial mesoderm which is continuous laterally with intermediate mesoderm and through that with the lateral mesoderm, the yolk sac and amniotic mesoderm.

At about Day 20 the paraxial mesoderm divides into paired blocks of somites. The first 38 pairs of somites are formed between Days 20–30 but eventually 42–44 pairs are formed. Each block has a cavity or myocoele which quickly disappears. The ventromedial part (sclerotome) of each somite will differentiate into vertebrae and ribs. The dorsolateral part (dermomyotome) will give rise to skeletal muscles and the dermal layer of the skin.

35c. Stage 17 (Day 41). Somites persist in the region of the tail as blocks of mesoderm. 12 mm CR

36. Stage 15 (Day 33). A transverse section through the lumbar region. 8 mm CR

36 from LHSM

1. amnion
2. arm bud
3. chorionic villi
4. cord (umbilical)
5. eye
6. hindbrain
7. leg bud
8. liver
9. neural tube
10. somite
11. tail

Coelom

Spaces appearing in the lateral plate and cardiogenic mesoderm of the primitive streak embryo coalesce to form the horseshoe-shaped intraembryonic coelom. The mesoderm is divided into two sheets; a somatic layer adjacent to the embryonic ectoderm and continuous with the mesoderm covering the amnion; and a splanchnic layer adjacent to the endoderm and continuous with the mesoderm covering the yolk sac.

The pericardial cavity will form in the curved portion of the horseshoe, while the two straight portions become the pleural and peritoneal cavities. At the lateral edges of the embryo the cavities are continuous with the extraembryonic coelom.

As the head, tail, and lateral folds of the embryo form, the future mouth (prochordal plate oral membrane) and cloacal membrane are carried ventrally. The horseshoe-shaped coelom is also carried on to the ventral aspect. As the head fold forms, the future pericardial cavity is carried beneath the foregut, where it expands around the developing heart to form the pericardial cavity. Caudal to the pericardial cavity the coelom on each side narrows and each is called a pericardio–peritoneal canal. These two narrow canals connect the pericardial cavity with the two abdominal parts of the coelom.

The two peritoneal cavities become a single cavity, except in the region of the caudal foregut. During Week 10 the peritoneal cavity is separated from the extraembryonic coelom at the umbilicus as the intestines return to the abdomen (see Midgut rotation).

37. Approximately Stages 10–11 (Days 22–24). A transverse section of the embryo and embryonic membranes.

1.	amnion
2.	extraembryonic coelom
3.	neural tube
4.	yolk sac cavity

DIVISIONS OF THE COELOM

Four partitions form, one at each end of the two pericardio–peritoneal canals, so separating the pericardial cavity from the pleural cavities and the pleural cavities from the peritoneal cavities.

The partition between pericardial and pleural cavities is formed as the lung buds grow (see Lungs). They expand and press adjacent mesoderm into the pericardio–peritoneal canals. The mesoderm covering the lung buds forms visceral pleura, while the outer mesodermal wall of the coelom becomes parietal pleura.

The common cardinal veins further narrow the pericardio–peritoneal canals when they become invested with a ridge of mesoderm (pleuro-pericardial membrane).

As the lungs expand further, the pleural cavities extend around the heart ventrally and split the mesoderm into two layers: fibrous pericardium and body wall.

With the descent of the heart, growth of the common cardinal veins, and formation of the pleural cavities, the pleuro-pericardial membranes fuse in Week 7 with mesoderm ventral to the esophagus.

The pleuro-peritoneal membranes divide the pleural cavities and peritoneal cavity. These membranes form as the pleural cavities expand to extend around the heart. They grow medially and ventrally, and in Week 6 their free edges fuse with the septum transversum and dorsal mesentery of the esophagus. With the extension of muscle into these membranes and the increase in liver size the pleuro-peritoneal openings are closed.

Germ Layer Derivatives

ECTODERM DERIVATIVES

Surface ectoderm
epidermis, hair, nails, sweat glands, sebaceous glands, mammary glands, lens of eye, inner ear, enamel of teeth, and anterior pituitary

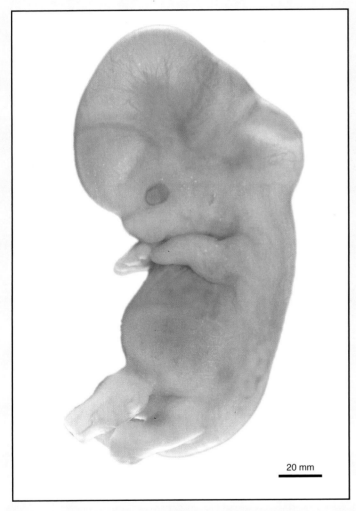

20 mm

38. Stage 19 (Days 47–48). The arms curve over the heart bulge and the toe rays are present on the foot. 20 mm CR

Neuroectoderm
Neural tube
central nervous system, retina, pineal body, and posterior pituitary

Neural crest
cranial and spinal sensory nerves and ganglia, adrenal medulla, pigment cells, head mesoderm, branchial arch cartilages, sympathetic ganglia and nerves, and Schwann cells

ENDODERM DERIVATIVES

Epithelial parts of the tonsils, pharynx, thyroid, parathyroids, pharyngotympanic tube, tympanic cavity, trachea, bronchi, and lungs. Epithelium of gastrointestinal tract, liver, pancreas, urachus, and urinary bladder

MESODERM DERIVATIVES

Head
skull, dentin, muscles, and connective tissue

Paraxial
skeleton (except skull), muscles of trunk, dermis of skin, and connective tissue

Intermediate
urogenital system (gonads, ducts, and accessory glands)

Lateral plate
cardiovascular system, blood cells, lymphatic system and cells of lymph, spleen, adrenal cortex, visceral and limb muscles, visceral connective tissue, serous membranes of pericardium, pleura, and peritoneum

Fetal Membranes and Placenta

The embryonic (and fetal) membranes and the placenta protect the embryo (and fetus), providing for nutrition, respiration and excretion, and hormone production during development. These membranes are the amnion, chorion, allantois, and yolk sac; they are formed by the zygote. The placenta forms from the fetal chorion and from the maternal endometrium. At birth the umbilical cord, placenta, amnion, and chorion are expelled after the fetus as 'afterbirth' (see Childbirth.)

As the blastocyst implants in the maternal endometrium (Days 7–10), a decidual reaction occurs. The stromal cells enlarge and increase in number. The glands and blood vessels also respond. Three regions develop in the decidua in relation to the implantation site; the area overlying the conceptus is the *decidua capsularis*; the area underlying the conceptus is the *decidua basalis*; and the remainder of the maternal mucosa is the *decidua parietalis*.

Chorion

Between Days 13 and 14 the cytotrophoblast proliferates to form clumps that extend into the syncytiotrophoblast. These are the primary chorionic villi which soon branch. At about Day 15 the villi acquire connective tissue cores and are then called secondary villi. They cover the entire surface of the chorion. Capillaries develop in the villi (tertiary villi). All three types of villi may be present at the same time. Cytotrophoblast extensions from the villi penetrate the syncytiotrophoblast layer and join to form the cytotrophoblastic shell which anchors the chorionic sac to the maternal endometrium. Between Weeks 5–10 growth of the chorionic sac is very rapid.

Up to Week 8 the chorionic sac is covered with villi. But as the sac grows, the blood vessels in the *decidua capsularis* are compressed, and degenerate; the chorion in this region becomes smooth (*chorion laeve*). At the same time, the villi in the *decidua basalis* increase to form the *chorion frondosum* (the fetal component of the placenta). The *decidua basalis* forms the maternal component (decidual plate). As the villi invade the *decidua basalis* they leave decidual tissue wedges, called placental septa, which divide the fetal part of the placenta into 10–38 cotyledons, each of which contains two or more main stem villi.

As the fetus grows the *decidua capsularis* extends into the uterine cavity and eventually contacts and fuses with the *decidua parietalis*. By Week 22 the *decidua capsularis* degenerates owing to a reduced blood supply.

- Chorionic villus sampling: from Week 7 biopsies of chorionic villi can be obtained by inserting a hollow needle through the vagina and uterus or through the maternal abdominal wall. Ultrasound can be used to guide the needle. Limb abnormalities have been associated with this technique.

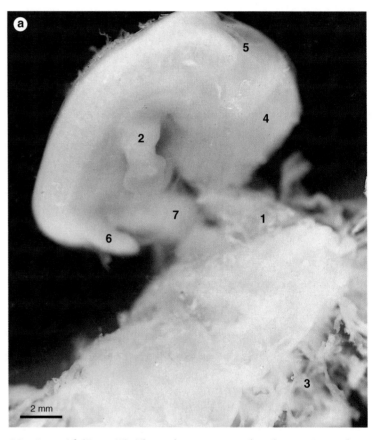

39a. Stage 16 (Days 37). The embryo connected to the amnion and chorion by the umbilical cord. 12 mm CR

39b. A higher magnification of the chorionic villi of the embryo in **39a**.

1. amnion
2. arm bud
3. chorionic villi
4. head
5. hindbrain
6. leg bud
7. umbilical cord

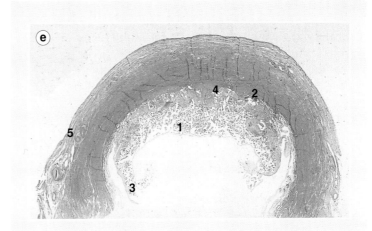

39c. The chorionic sac (approximately 26 mm in diameter) of a Stage 12 embryo.

1. amnion
2. chorion laeve
3. chorionic villi
4. embryonic surface
5. umbilical vessels

39d. The chorionic sac opened to show the amnion, umbilical cord, and vessels. The vessels have been injected with colored media.

39e. A transverse section through the placenta of a 15 mm CR embryo *in situ.*

1. chorionic villi
2. *decidua basalis*
3. *decidua capsularis*
4. *decidua parietalis*
5. myometrium

39d and **39e** *from the W.J. Hamilton Collection*

40a. Week 9. The fetus *in situ* in the chorionic sac. 46 mm CR ♂

40b. The fetus in **40a** with the chorionic sac opened. The amnion is present, but is transparent. 46 mm CR ♂

1. amnion	3. eye	5. leg	7. umbilical cord
2. chorionic villi	4. head	6. smooth chorion	

Amnion

The amniotic cavity forms when spaces in the inner cell mass and trophoblast coalesce to form a cavity above the embryonic disc ectoderm. The epithelial roof forms from cytotrophoblast cells and its outer surface becomes covered with extraembryonic mesoderm. As the extraembryonic coelom extends, it separates the amniotic cavity from the chorion except in the region of the embryonic (connecting) stalk. When the embryo forms head and tail folds the amnion is carried around to the ventral side of the embryo.

The amniotic cavity enlarges at the expense of the extraembryonic coelom, which gradually disappears. The amnion lines the chorion, which fuses first with the *decidua capsularis* and then with the *decidua parietalis*, except in the region of the body stalk where it follows and lines the outer surface of the connecting stalk (later the umbilical cord).

The amniotic cavity initially contains fluid produced by its cellular walls, but the majority comes from maternal blood and in late pregnancy 500 ml of fetal urine is excreted daily into the cavity. The amniotic fluid physically cushions the embryo, acts as a barrier to infection, maintains a constant temperature, prevents the amnion from adhering to the developing embryo, and permits symmetrical growth and free movements of the fetus which assist muscular development and normal lung development.

By Week 37 about 1000 ml of amniotic fluid is present; the fetus swallows and absorbs about 400 ml per day, and it produces 500 ml of urine daily back into the cavity. The water in the amniotic fluid is changed every 3 h via the amniochorionic membrane.

The amniotic fluid contains desquamated fetal epithelial cells, lanugo, *vernix caseosa*, proteins, fats, carbohydrates, hormones, enzymes, pigments, fetal urine and 98–99% water.

At term, a dilatation of amnion and chorion filled with amniotic fluid is present in the dilating cervix (see Childbirth).

- Amniocentesis: from about Week 14, amniotic fluid can be sampled by inserting a hollow needle through the maternal abdominal wall, the uterus, and into the amniotic cavity. Ultrasound can be used to guide the needle.
- Excessive quantities of amniotic fluid (polyhydramnios) and insufficient quantities (oligohydramnios) may be present in association with fetal abnormalities. These conditions may be diagnosed by ultrasonography.
- Occasionally, the amnion does not rupture at birth and the neonate is born enclosed in the amniotic sac or 'caul'.

41b. Week 8. The embryo suspended in the amniotic sac. 31 mm CR

41b from RFHSM

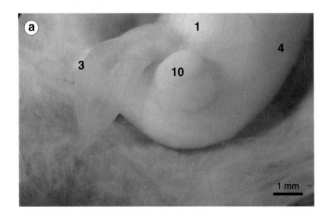

41a. Stages 17 (Days 41). The early embryonic stalk is covered with a tube of amnion which is continuous with the amnion in contact with the chorion. 12 mm CR

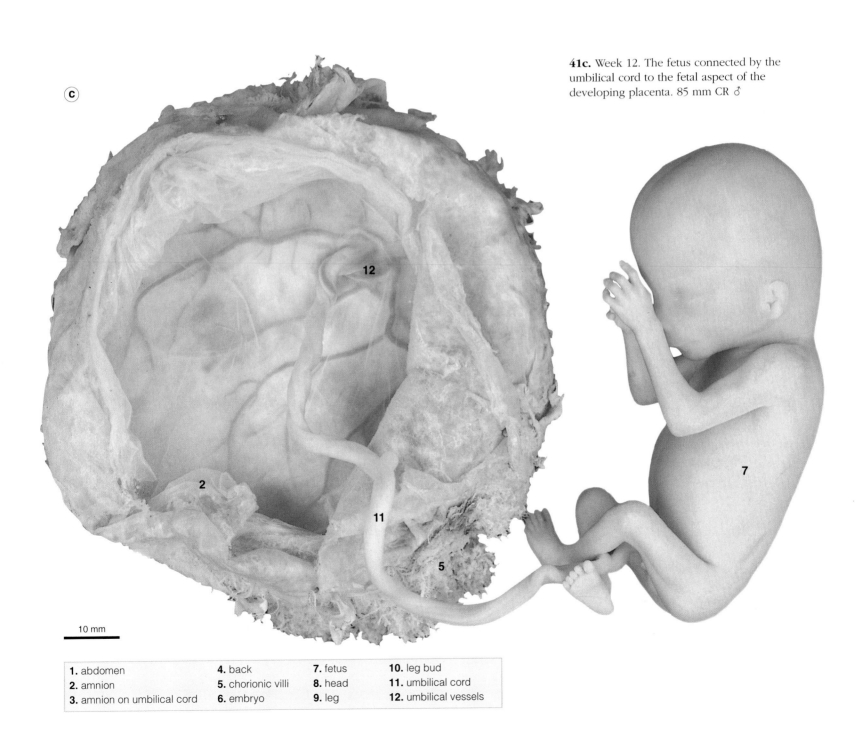

41c. Week 12. The fetus connected by the umbilical cord to the fetal aspect of the developing placenta. 85 mm CR ♂

10 mm

1. abdomen	**4.** back	**7.** fetus	**10.** leg bud
2. amnion	**5.** chorionic villi	**8.** head	**11.** umbilical cord
3. amnion on umbilical cord	**6.** embryo	**9.** leg	**12.** umbilical vessels

Yolk sac

1. amnion
2. chorionic villi
3. fetal surface of placenta
4. head
5. ribs
6. toes
7. umbilical blood vessels
8. umbilical cord
9. yolk sac
10. yolk sac and stalk

42a. Stage 13 (Day 28). The early yolk sac. 4–6 mm CR

42a and *42b* from the *W.J. Hamilton Collection*

42b. Stage 23 (Days 56–57). The yolk sac and stalk. 28–30 mm CR

10 mm

42c. Week 9. The yolk sac is shrunken. 44 mm CR

5 mm

The primary yolk sac is lined by a thin exocoelomic (Heuser's) membrane. As the extraembryonic coelom forms the primary yolk sac degenerates and a smaller secondary yolk sac forms lined by endoderm. The first vascular blood forms from yolk sac mesoderm (Week 3). This will provide embryonic blood until the liver starts to form blood (Week 6). It also provides nutrients during Weeks 2 and 3 while the chorioallantoic placenta develops. During Week 3 the primordial germ cells formed on the yolk sac migrate into the embryo. In Week 4 the body folds constrict the yolk sac and the portion incorporated into the embryo forms the epithelium of the gut tube. The extraembryonic portion is the yolk sac remnant. The gut tube is divided into foregut, midgut, and hindgut. The embryonic foregut includes the pharynx and its derivatives, the lower respiratory tract, esophagus, stomach, liver, pancreas, biliary apparatus, and the duodenum to the entrance of the common bile duct. The celiac artery supplies all but the pharynx, respiratory tract, and upper esophagus.

The embryonic midgut includes the small intestines from the entrance of the common bile duct, the cecum, and the vermiform appendix, and the ascending and proximal part of the transverse colon. The superior mesenteric artery supplies the midgut.

The embryonic hindgut includes the distal part of the transverse colon, descending and sigmoid colon, rectum, upper anal canal, and part of the urogenital system. The inferior mesenteric artery supplies the hindgut.

In Week 10 the yolk sac remnant (stalk) detaches from the gut (see Midgut rotation) and by Week 12 it is shrunken and hardened.

- The yolk sac is visible by ultrasound examination from Week 5 until 11 weeks gestation.

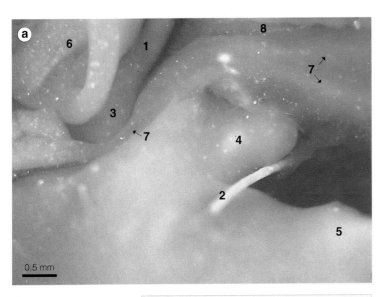

43a. Stage 19 (Days 47–48). The developing urinary bladder and allantois. The umbilical cord has been dissected open. 20 mm CR

1. allantois
2. cactus needle
3. developing urinary bladder (urogenital sinus)
4. genital tubercle
5. leg bud
6. midgut and hindgut
7. umbilical artery
8. umbilical cord dissected open

Allantois

The allantois appears on Day 16 as a diverticulum of the yolk sac. Between Weeks 3–5 blood forms in the walls of the allantois. The umbilical vein and arteries form from its blood vessels, and amniotic cavity fluid enters the fetal circulation via the umbilical vein. This is eventually then transferred to the maternal blood.

The intraembryonic portion of the allantois extends from the umbilicus to the urinary bladder. As the bladder forms, the allantois becomes the urachus (see Urinary bladder). During Weeks 5–8 the extraembryonic portion degenerates.

- In the infant, the urachus becomes fibrous and forms the median umbilical ligament.

43b. Week 11. The urachus, viewed from the ventral surface. 65 mm CR ♂

1. anterior abdominal wall (cut)
2. left umbilical artery
3. leg
4. penis
5. testis
6. umbilical cord
7. urachus
8. urinary bladder

Placenta

The placenta is interposed between fetal and maternal circulations and has several functions; these include metabolism and transfer of nutrients, wastes, antibodies, hormones, and electrolytes. Drugs and infectious organisms may also cross the placenta. The placenta is a source of hormones.

The placental membrane is composed of syncytiotrophoblast, cytotrophoblast, a connective tissue core in each villus, and fetal capillary endothelium. Macrophage-like Hofbauer cells appear in the cores of villi in early pregnancy.

The villous tree grows by repeatedly branching and the fetal capillaries increase in number and size. In this way an initially terminal villus can become an intermediate villus. Eventually, the capillaries come to lie close to the syncytiotrophoblast, as the placental membrane becomes thinner in late pregnancy.

THE MATURE PLACENTA

The mature placenta is discoidal and flattened in shape; it weighs approximately 500 g at birth. It is about 20 cm in diameter and 2.5 cm thick at the center. Implantation is usually in the upper part of the uterus on the dorsal aspect.

The fetal surface of the placenta is smooth with the umbilical cord attached near the center. The chorionic vessels are visible through the amnion as they ramify in the chorionic mesoderm (chorionic plate).

The maternal oriented surface of the placenta is rough and raised into 10–38 cotyledons. Grooves between the cotyledons mark the site of the placental septa.

The amnion and chorion are continuous with the edges of the placenta. At parturition, the umbilical cord, placenta, amnion, and chorion follow the fetus as the 'afterbirth'.

- If implantation occurs in the lower uterus, the placenta may cover the internal os *(placenta previa)* and obstruct the fetus during parturition.
- Implantation may occur outside the uterus in an ectopic site [abdominal cavity, or uterine (Fallopian) tubes].
- Ectopic pregnancy is a life-threatening condition.

44a. Week 23. Section of a placenta from a fetus. 220 mm CR ♂

1. chorionic vessels
2. fetal surface
3. maternal surface
4. placental septa

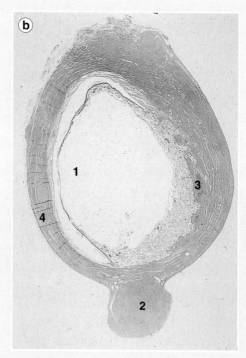

44b. A transverse histological section of the placenta *in situ*. 30 mm CR embryo

***44b** from the W.J. Hamilton Collection*

1. amniotic cavity
2. cervix
3. placenta
4. myometrium of uterus

45a. A radiograph of a placenta and fetus injected with chromopaque. 30 mm foot length.

1.	chorionic artery
2.	cotyledonary artery
3.	fetus
4.	placenta
5.	umbilical cord
6.	umbilical arteries
7.	uterus

45a from Mr J. Bashford, J.D. Boyd

45b from the W.J. Hamilton Collection

45b. A radiograph of the placenta of a 140 mm CR fetus injected with chromopaque.

45c. A radiograph of a placenta *in utero* of a 170 mm CR fetus (on page 111) injected with chromopaque.

45c from Mr J. Bashford, W.J. Hamilton and J.D. Boyd Collections

46a from RCOG

46a. The placenta of uniovular twins.

Multiple births

Twins arise from either a single, fertilized oocyte which divides into two masses (monozygotic, identical, or like twins) or two separate oocytes are fertilized (dizygotic, fraternal, or unlike twins).

The amnion, chorion, and placenta of monozygotic or identical twins reflect when the single fertilized oocyte divides into two masses. There may be two amnions, two chorions, and two placentae (which may fuse). Other combinations include two amnions, one chorion, and one placenta; and one amnion, one chorion, and one placenta. Dizygotic or unlike twins have two amnions, two chorions, and two placentae which may fuse.

Triplets may arise from one, two, or three fertilized oocytes. Quadruplets may arise from one, two, three, or four fertilized oocytes.

- Multiple births may result when several pre-embryos are returned after *in vitro* fertilization.
- Superovulation can result in multiple births.
- There is an increased incidence of fetal abnormalities in multiple births.

46b and **46c.** The placentae of triplets and quadruplets.

46b from the W.J. Hamilton Collection

46b. The placenta of female triplets. Three amnions and a single chorion are present. Several anastomoses are present between the three circulations. The chorionic vessels have been injected with red, blue, and yellow resin.

46c from RCOG

46c. The placenta of quadruplets.

1. amniochorion
2. amnion
3. fetal surface
4. placenta (fetal surface)
5. umbilical cord

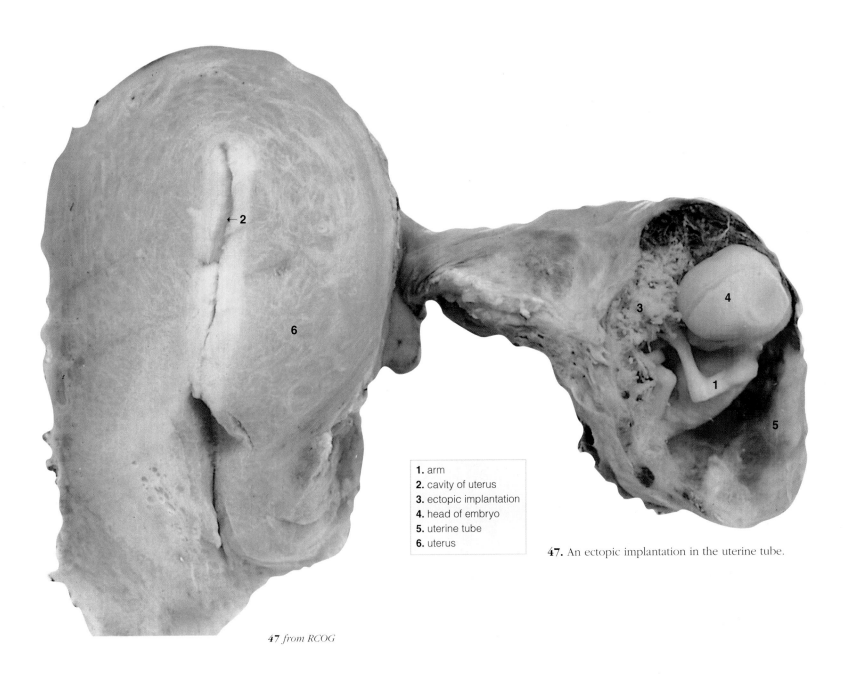

1. arm
2. cavity of uterus
3. ectopic implantation
4. head of embryo
5. uterine tube
6. uterus

47. An ectopic implantation in the uterine tube.

47 from RCOG

Umbilical cord

The early embryo has a very thick embryonic stalk (body, connecting, or umbilical stalk) containing two umbilical arteries, two umbilical veins, the allantois, and primary mesoderm cells. The arteries carry blood from the embryo to the chorionic villi and the umbilical veins return blood to the embryo. The right umbilical vein degenerates.

In Week 5 the amnion expands to fill the entire extraembryonic coelom. This process forces the yolk stalk against the embryonic stalk and covers the entire contents with a tube of amniotic ectoderm, so forming the umbilical cord. The cord is narrower in diameter than the embryonic stalk and it rapidly increases in length. The connective tissue in the umbilical cord is called Wharton's jelly and is derived from the primary mesoderm cells. The umbilical vein and two arteries twist around one another. The early umbilical cord starts to twist spirally on itself. It is not uncommon to find the cord looped around the fetus. In Weeks 35–38 the attachment of the umbilical cord becomes central in the abdomen.

- At birth the mature cord is about 54 cm in length and 12 mm in diameter. There may be as many as 40 spiral twists present in the cord, as well as false knots (irregular projections of blood vessels) and true knots (the fetus has moved through a loop of cord).
- When the blood flow is interrupted at birth some of the intraembryonic parts of the umbilical arteries and vein gradually become fibrous cords.
- The course of the left umbilical vein is discernible in the adult as a fibrous cord from the umbilicus to the liver (*ligamentum teres*) contained within the falciform ligament.
- The umbilical arteries are retained proximally as the internal iliac arteries and give off the superior vesical arteries, and distally as the medial umbilical ligaments within the medial umbilical folds to the umbilicus.
- The umbilical cord remains stiff during development because of the blood flowing through it.
- The normal regression of the cord stump may be an important medico-legal factor in determining infant survival time.

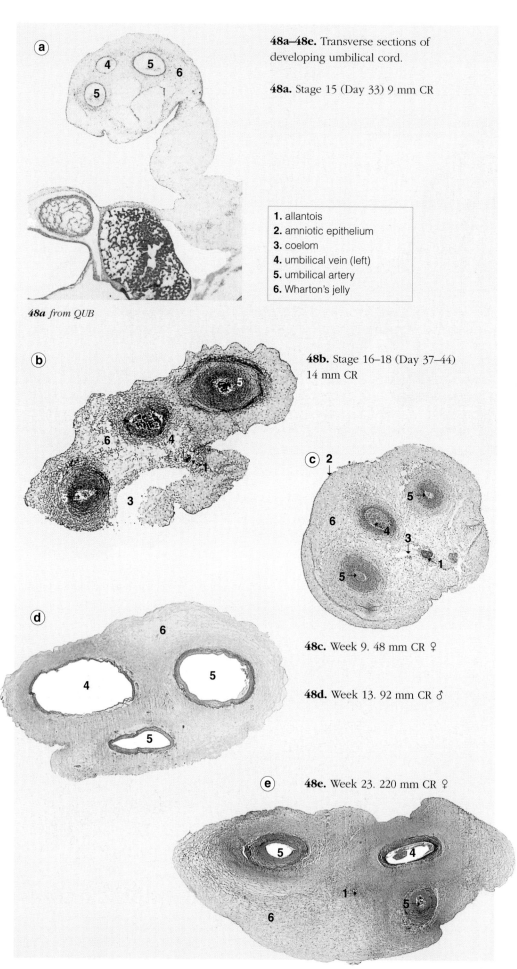

48a–48e. Transverse sections of developing umbilical cord.

48a. Stage 15 (Day 33) 9 mm CR

1. allantois
2. amniotic epithelium
3. coelom
4. umbilical vein (left)
5. umbilical artery
6. Wharton's jelly

48a *from QUB*

48b. Stage 16–18 (Day 37–44) 14 mm CR

48c. Week 9. 48 mm CR ♀

48d. Week 13. 92 mm CR ♂

48e. Week 23. 220 mm CR ♀

48f. Full-term umbilical vessels injected with plastic resin. Umbilical arteries are blue and the vein is red.

48g. Arteriograph of the umbilical vessels of a placenta of a 135 mm CR fetus.

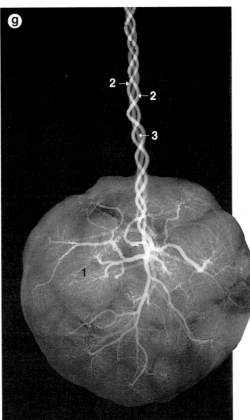

1. placenta (fetal surface)
2. umbilical arteries
3. umbilical vein

48f from D. Adams and I. Indams

48g from Mr J. Bashford, J.D. Boyd

49a–49j. Development of the umbilical cord

49a. Stage 17 (Day 41). 12 mm CR

49b. Stage 17 (Day 41). 12 mm CR

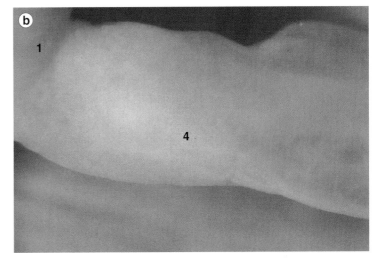

1. abdomen
2. arm bud
3. leg bud
4. umbilical cord

49c. Stages 16–18 (Days 37–44).
14 mm CR

49c from RCS

49d. Week 8. 39 mm CR

49e. Week 10. 60 mm CR ♀

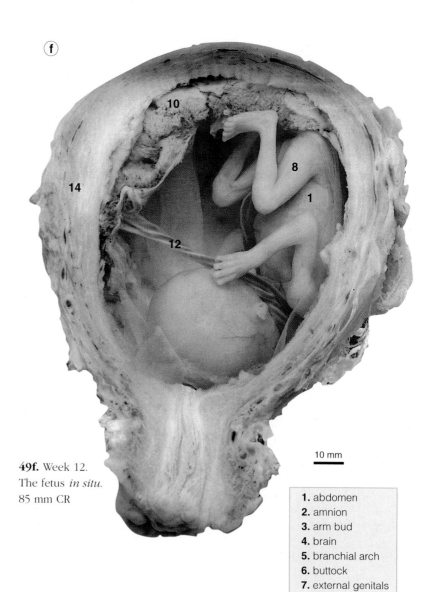

49f. Week 12.
The fetus *in situ.*
85 mm CR

49g. Week 15. 130 mm CR ♀

1. abdomen
2. amnion
3. arm bud
4. brain
5. branchial arch
6. buttock
7. external genitals
8. leg
9. leg bud
10. placenta
11. spiral twist
12. umbilical cord
13. umbilical vessels
14. uterus

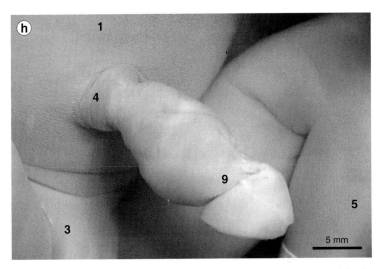

49h. Week 15. Continuation of the amniotic cord epithelium and fetal epidermis. 130 mm CR ♀

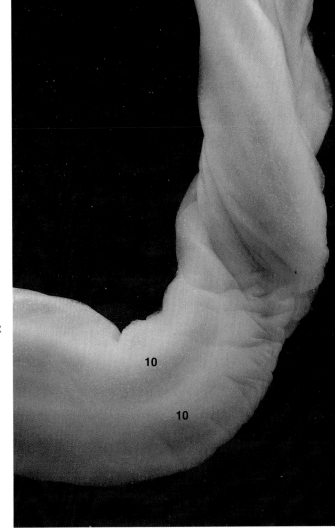

49i. Week 22. 210 mm CR

49j. Week 35. The umbilical cord. ♀

1. abdomen
2. arm
3. external genitals
4. fetal epidermis
5. leg
6. plastic clamp
7. thorax
8. umbilical cord
9. umbilical cord covered with amnion
10. umbilical vessels

50a and **50b.** Stage 19 (Days 47–48). The course of one umbilical artery to the umbilical cord. 20 mm CR

1. diaphragm
2. external oblique muscle
3. falciform ligament
4. genital tubercle
5. herniated midgut
6. inferior epigastric vessels
7. internal oblique muscle
8. internal thoracic artery
9. intestine
10. left lobe of liver
11. left umbilical vein
12. leg bud
13. red cactus needle
14. ribs
15. right lobe of liver
16. right lobe of liver removed
17. transversus abdominus muscle
18. umbilical artery
19. umbilical cord
20. umbilical vein
21. urinary bladder

50b. The same embryo as in **50a**, but with the umbilical cord dissected away. 20 mm CR

50c. Week 10. The course of the umbilical vein from the umbilical cord, viewed from the right. 56 mm CR

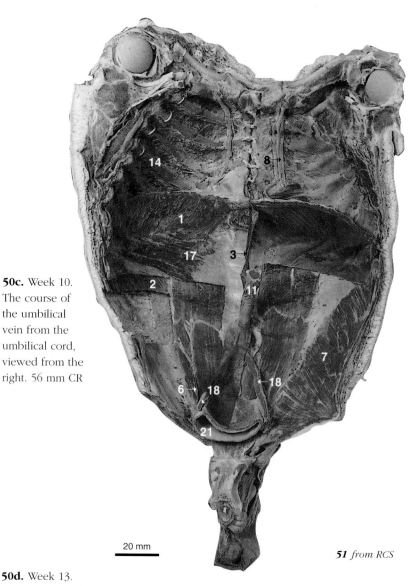

50d. Week 13. Anterior view of the liver. 92 mm CR ♀

51. The anterior thoracic and abdominal wall in a full-term fetus. View from behind. Peritoneum and parts of muscles and the rectus sheaths have been removed.

51 from RCS

Head and Neck Development

Brain

The first rudiment of the nervous system is the midline ectoderm neural plate (Week 3). Neural folds form which rise and fuse to form a tube starting in the region between the brain and spinal cord. Fusion proceeds both cranially and caudally leaving both ends open; these are the rostral (anterior) and caudal (posterior) neuropores. The pores will eventually close. The *lamina terminalis* forms the cephalic end of the neural tube when the anterior neuropore closes. The main divisions of the central nervous system are established at this stage (Week 4): forebrain, midbrain, hindbrain, and spinal cord. The optic cup is an outgrowth of the forebrain. In Week 5 the forebrain (prosencephalon) divides into the telencephalon, the rostral forebrain, with the primordia of the cerebral hemispheres and the caudal forebrain called the diencephalon. The midbrain (or mesencephalon) remains as before, but the hindbrain (or rhombencephalon) forms two regions: the metencephalon and myelencephalon.

CAVITIES OF THE BRAIN

A pair of cerebral vesicles grows out from the median part of the telencephalon. The hollow space in each cerebral hemisphere is called the lateral ventricle, which is continuous with the third ventricle (the original forebrain cavity) via the interventricular foramen. The third ventricle is continuous with the wide lumen of the midbrain, the cerebral aqueduct, which is continuous with the hindbrain lumen through a constriction, the isthmus. The diamond-shaped hindbrain's fourth ventricle merges into the central canal of the spinal cord without a distinct boundary.

FLEXURES

Three flexures appear in the brain due to unequal growth. The first, the midbrain flexure, appears during Week 4 when the forebrain bends in a ventral direction. The second flexure, the cervical or neck flexure, occurs between the hindbrain and spinal cord. This flexure diminishes and eventually disappears after the head extends during Week 8 (see Neck).

The third flexure, the pontine flexure, occurs in the region of the pons (Week 5). It does not noticeably alter the outline of the head as the first two flexures do. It does, however, cause the rhombencephalon's lateral walls to splay and thin, so that the roof forms a diamond shape. The flexure divides the rhombencephalon into the metencephalon and myelencephalon. The alar and basal laminae come to lie in the floor of the rhombencephalon with the *sulcus limitans* between the two.

LAYERS OF THE BRAIN

Initially, the brain and spinal cord have the same three layers; the ventricular, intermediate, and marginal layers. In the brain a

fourth layer is added when cells from the intermediate layer migrate through the marginal zone to the outside and form a layer of cortex. Therefore, gray matter (cortex) is on the outside of the brain and the axons from cell bodies pass centrally. This is unlike the spinal cord, where the axons pass peripherally.

52a and **52b**. Flexures of the brain.

52a. Stage 17 (Day 41). 12 mm CR

52b. Stage 19 (Days 47–48). The hindbrain roof has been removed. 20 mm CR

1. cervical flexure
2. eye
3. forebrain
4. heart
5. hindbrain
6. liver bulge
7. midbrain
8. midbrain flexure
9. pontine flexure
10. umbilical cord

FOREBRAIN

The forebrain has two lateral expansions, the cerebral (telencephalic) vesicles. The cavities of the cerebral vesicles are the lateral ventricles and these are continuous with the third ventricle. The telencephalon consists of the rostral forebrain, including the cerebral hemispheres. The diencephalon is the posterior part of the forebrain. The third ventricle is reduced by three swellings in its lateral walls; the epithalamus, thalamus, and hypothalamus. The two thalami expand and usually fuse in the midline. Two mamillary bodies form on the ventral surface of the hypothalamus. The pineal gland is a midline diverticulum of the diencephalic roof.

Telencephalon

The cerebral vesicles are originally in wide communication with the third ventricle via the interventricular foramina, although these openings are later reduced. The medial walls of the cerebral vesicles become very thin and are penetrated by vascular pia mater to form the choroid plexus at this site (choroid fissure). The cerebral hemispheres expand like two large balloons and cover the diencephalon, the midbrain, and, finally, the hindbrain. As the hemispheres meet in the midline they flatten medially and trap mesoderm which forms the falx cerebri. The caudal end of the hemisphere turns ventrally, and then cranially, to bury the insula and form the temporal lobe adjacent to the lateral sulcus. Thus, the cerebral hemisphere becomes 'C' shaped. The choroid fissue follows its line of growth.

In the floor of each hemisphere the corpus striatum develops and fibers passing to and from the cerebral cortex divide it into the caudate and lentiform nuclei (Week 6). This fiber pathway (internal capsule) becomes 'C' shaped.

As the cerebral hemispheres grow, several groups of fibers (or commissures) connect the corresponding areas of the two hemispheres; these are the anterior commissure, the hippocampal (fornix) commissure, the corpus callosum, and the optic chiasma.

The surface of the hemispheres is smooth until Weeks 25 and 26 when sulci and gyri develop and the brain volume is increased.

53a–53c. Stages 16–17 (Days 37–41). Forebrain development. 12 mm CR

| 1. branchial arch |
| 2. eye |
| 3. forebrain |
| 4. hindbrain |
| 5. liver shadow |
| 6. midbrain |
| 7. umbilical cord |

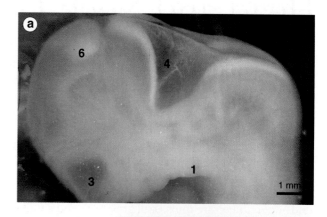

53a. Note the diamond-shaped hindbrain and lateral vesicles of the forebrain, viewed from the left.

53b. The same embryo as in **53a** seen by transmitted light, viewed from the right and front.

53c. Lateral view of the same embryo as in **53a**, viewed from the right.

53d. Stage 17 (Day 41). Lateral view of the developing cerebral vesicles. 14 mm CR

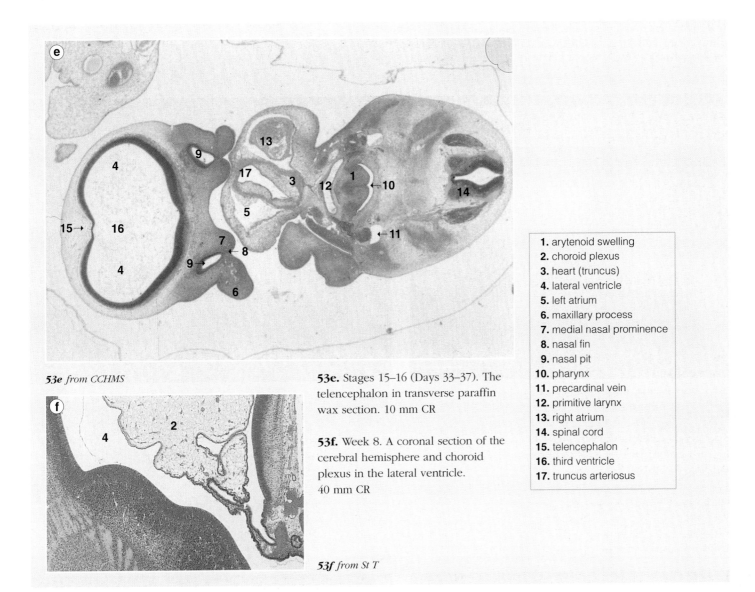

53e from CCHMS

53e. Stages 15–16 (Days 33–37). The telencephalon in transverse paraffin wax section. 10 mm CR

53f. Week 8. A coronal section of the cerebral hemisphere and choroid plexus in the lateral ventricle. 40 mm CR

53f from St T

1. arytenoid swelling
2. choroid plexus
3. heart (truncus)
4. lateral ventricle
5. left atrium
6. maxillary process
7. medial nasal prominence
8. nasal fin
9. nasal pit
10. pharynx
11. precardinal vein
12. primitive larynx
13. right atrium
14. spinal cord
15. telencephalon
16. third ventricle
17. truncus arteriosus

54a and **54b.** Stage 19 (Days 47–48). Blood supply to the developing brain. **54b** is a higher magnification of the midbrain in **54a**. 20 mm CR

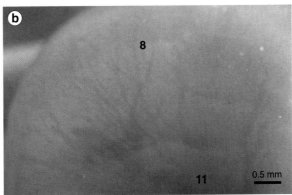

1. eye
2. forebrain
3. heart
4. hindbrain
5. internal jugular vein
6. mandible
7. maxilla
8. midbrain
9. sigmoid sinus
10. superior sagittal sinus
11. transverse sinus

55a–55f. Development and rapid relative growth of the cerebral hemispheres, compared with the midbrain, and the development of the gyri. Note the straight central sulcus.

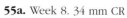

1. cerebellum
2. cerebral hemispheres (telencephalon)
3. frontal lobe
4. insula
5. lateral sulcus
6. medulla
7. mesencephalon
8. occipital lobe
9. parietal lobe
10. temporal lobe

55a. Week 8. 34 mm CR

55b. Week 8. 40 mm CR

55c. Week 10. 57 mm CR ♂

55d. Week 13. 101 mm CR ♀

55e. Week 18. 152 mm CR ♂

55f. Week 28.

55f from RFHSM

1. central sulcus
2. cerebellum
3. cerebral hemispheres (telencephalon)
4. gyri
5. lateral fissure
6. medulla
7. occipital lobe
8. parietal lobe
9. sulci
10. temporal lobe

56a and **56b.** The cranial cavity.

56a. Week 13. Viewed from above. Note the lack of frontal sinus. 101 mm CR ♀

56b. Week 24. The cranial cavity exposed from behind.

1. anterior cranial fossa
2. cribriform plate of the ethmoid and remains of the olfactory bulb
3. crista galli
4. hand
5. medulla
6. middle cranial fossa
7. optic canal
8. posterior cranial fossa
9. sella turcica (pituitary fossa with pituitary gland)
10. shoulder
11. spinal cord
12. spinal ganglia

56b from RFHSM

57a–57d. Cerebral hemispheres overgrowing the midbrain, viewed from above (superior or cranial surface).

1. cerebellum
2. cerebral hemispheres
3. falx cerebri
4. hindbrain
5. mesencephalon
6. spinal cord

57a. Week 8. 34 mm CR

57b. Week 10. 57 mm CR ♂

57c. Week 13. Note the smooth surface of the cerebral hemispheres. 101 mm CR ♀

57d. Week 18. The blood vessels are enlarged in this fetus. 152 mm CR ♂

58a–58d. The fetal brain at various stages of development, viewed from below.

1. anterior cerebral artery
2. basilar artery
3. cerebellum
4. frontal lobe
5. internal carotid artery
6. medulla
7. olfactory bulb
8. optic chiasma
9. pituitary stalk (cut)
10. pons
11. temporal lobe

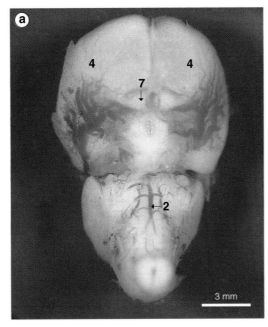

58a. Week 8. 34 mm CR

58b. Week 10. 57 mm CR ♂

58c. Week 13. 101 mm CR ♀

58d. Week 18. 152 mm CR ♂

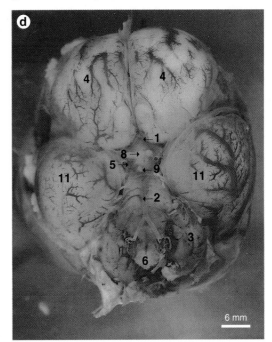

59a and **59b.** Stage 17 (Day 41). The midbrain in the 12 mm CR embryo.

1. back
2. branchial arches
3. forebrain
4. heart
5. hindbrain roof
6. midbrain

59a. Viewed from the left.

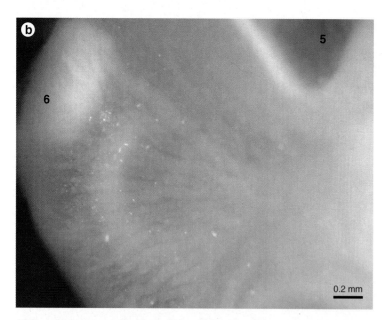

59b. A higher magnification of the midbrain in **59a**.

MIDBRAIN

The midbrain is most prominent at the midbrain flexure. Caudally it is constricted at the isthmus. Rostrally, its wide lumen is the mesocoele and its roof the smooth tectum. It joins the third and fourth ventricles. The lateral walls are divided into dorsal (or alar) and ventral (or basal) laminae.

The wide lumen is reduced to a narrow channel, the cerebral aqueduct, when four colliculi form in the tectum from neuroblasts in the alar laminae. The walls are thickened laterally and ventrally by the formation of the red nucleus, the nuclei of cranial nerves III and IV and reticular nuclei. The cerebral peduncles and substantia nigra also reduce the lumen of the aqueduct.

60a–60e. Hemisection (sagittal section) of the developing brain to illustrate sequentially the internal changes.

60a. Week 8. 34 mm CR

3 mm

60b. Week 10. Left brain. 57 mm CR ♂

5 mm

1. cerebellum
2. cerebral peduncles
3. corpora quadrigemina
4. corpus striatum
5. diencephalon
6. falx cerebri
7. hypophysis
8. mamillary body
9. medulla oblongata
10. mesencephalon
11. myelencephalon
12. occipital lobe
13. olfactory bulb
14. pineal body
15. pons
16. posterior commissure
17. telencephalon
18. thalamus

60c. Week 13. Left brain. 101 mm CR ♀

5 mm

60d. Week 18. Left brain. 152 mm CR ♂

10 mm

60e. The right side of the brain specimen in **60b**. The falx cerebri remains *in situ*.

3 mm

61a–61b. Week 8. Higher magnification of the hemisected brain in **60b**. 34 mm CR

1 mm

1. mamillary body
2. olfactory bulb
3. optic nerve
4. pituitary
5. telencephalon
6. thalamus

1 mm

62. Stage 16 (Day 37). The rhombomeres are visible.

1. branchial arch
2. hindbrain
3. rhombomere

HINDBRAIN

The diamond-shaped hindbrain (rhomb-encephalon) is continuous with the spinal cord. The pontine flexure divides the hindbrain into two parts; metencephalon (cephalically) and myelencephalon (caudally). The roof is very thin and the floor is thrown into a series of waves (rhombomeres), which later disappear. The cavity is the fourth ventricle and the central canal of the lower medulla. The otocyst lies caudal to the widest part of the diamond-shape of the hindbrain. The isthmus (from the midbrain) forms the anterior medullary velum, the superior cerebellar peduncles, and the cranial part of the fourth ventricle.

The metencephalon roof thickens to form the cerebellum and the floor becomes the pons. The middle part of the fourth ventricle is of metencephalic origin.

The floor of the myelencephalon contributes to the medulla oblongata, and in Weeks 14–17 the pyramids are formed by the downgrowing corticospinal fibers from the telencephalon. Its lumen is the caudal part of the fourth ventricle. The alar and basal laminae, separated by the sulcus limitans, are clearly distinguishable.

The choroid plexus invaginates into the roof. As cerebrospinal fluid (CSF) is formed by the choroid plexus, pressure increases in the fourth ventricle and three foramina form in the thin roof; the median foramen of Magendie, and the two paired lateral foramina of Luschka. These allow the CSF to escape into the subarachnoid space.

- If the aqueducts or foramina of Magendie or Luschka are blocked by scar tissue from intrauterine infection, the CSF cannot escape and congenital hydrocephalus results.

Cranial nerves

The olfactory (I) and optic (II) nerves are atypical in origin as they are extensions of the brain. The remaining cranial nerves can be divided into those with ganglia, i.e., having some sensory and/or autonomic components (V, VII, IX, and X) and those without ganglia. Sensory and autonomic cranial nerve ganglia form from neural crest similar to the spinal dorsal root or sympathetic ganglia.

The remaining cranial nerves are without ganglia and have no sensory or autonomic fibers.

The cranial nerves are, therefore, either purely sensory, purely motor, or mixed, while all the spinal nerves are mixed.

63a–63c. Stage 17 (Day 41). The hindbrain. 12 mm CR

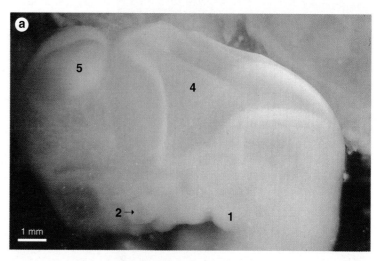

63a. Viewed from above left.

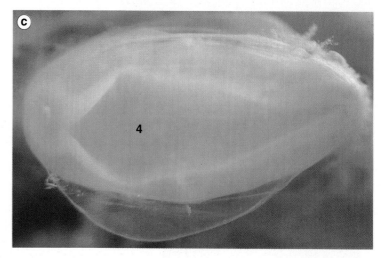

63b. The same embryo as in **63a**, viewed with transmitted light.

63c. Viewed from above.

1. branchial arch
2. eye (left)
3. forebrain
4. hindbrain
5. mesencephalon

64a and **64b.** Stage 18 (Day 41–44). The hindbrain viewed in sagittal section. 14 mm CR

1. neuromeres
2. pontine flexure
3. roof plate

64a. Right side of hindbrain.

64b. Left side of hindbrain in **64a**.

65a–65c. Stage 19 (Days 47–48). The midbrain and hindbrain viewed from the right. 20 mm CR

1. blood supply
2. choroid plexus
3. ear
4. eye (right)
5. hindbrain
6. midbrain

65b. A higher magnification of the hindbrain (medulla) in **65a**.

65c. A higher magnification of the hindbrain (cerebellum) in **65a**, viewed from the left.

66a and **66b.** Stage 19 (Days 47–48). The hindbrain viewed from above. The ectoderm and roof plate have been removed. 20 mm CR

1. cerebellum
2. entrance to aqueduct of mesencephalon
3. fourth ventricle
4. medulla

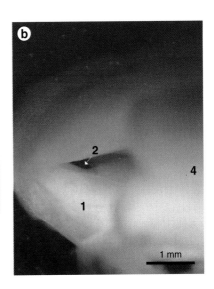

Cerebellum

The cerebellum develops as swellings formed from cells in the rhombic lip and dorsal part of the alar lamina of the metencephalon. Initially (Stages 15–16, Days 34–36), the swellings bulge into the fourth ventricle, fuse in the midline, enlarge externally at the expense of the interventricular portion, and overgrow the rostral half of the fourth ventricle, so overlapping the pons and medulla by Week 12. Transverse grooves appear on the dorsal aspect (Week 13) and the flocculonodular lobe is demarcated from the rest of the cerebellum.

67. Week 10. The hindbrain and developing cerebellum. 57 mm CR ♂

1. cerebellum
2. fourth ventricle with roof removed
3. mesencephalon

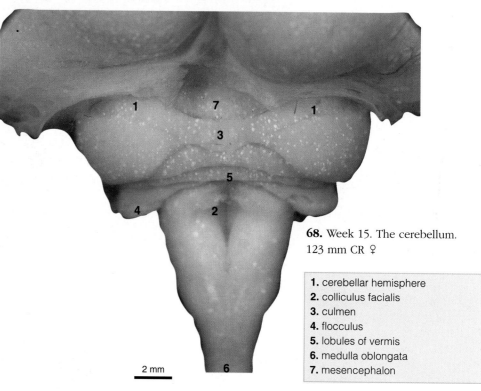

68. Week 15. The cerebellum. 123 mm CR ♀

1. cerebellar hemisphere
2. colliculus facialis
3. culmen
4. flocculus
5. lobules of vermis
6. medulla oblongata
7. mesencephalon

69a–69f. The development of the brain as seen in sagittal section.
69a. Week 16.
69b. Week 18.
69c. Week 19.

1. anterior cranial fossa
2. arm
3. body of mandible
4. cerebellar fossa
5. confluence of sinuses
6. dorsal
7. dorsum of tongue
8. esophagus
9. falx cerebri
10. hard palate
11. heart
12. intestines
13. leg
14. liver
15. nose
16. pituitary gland
17. sella turcica
18. soft palate
19. ventral
20. vertebrae

69a–69f from RCS

(d)

22
28
2
14
18
30
15
6
31
16

15 mm

69d. Week 19.

(e)

22
25
28
9
5

10 mm

69e. Week 19.

(f)

10
23
13
17
31

10 mm

69f. A higher magnification of **69c**.

1. anterior cranial fossa
2. arm
3. body of mandible
4. cerebellar fossa
5. confluence of sinuses
6. dorsal
7. dorsum of tongue
8. epiglottis
9. esophagus
10. falx cerebri
11. genioglossus muscle
12. geniohyoid muscle
13. hard palate
14. heart
15. intestines
16. leg
17. lip
18. liver
19. middle cranial fossa
20. mylohyoid muscle
21. nasal septum
22. nose
23. pituitary gland
24. posterior nasal aperture (choana)
25. sella turcica
26. soft palate
27. tentorium cerebelli
28. tongue
29. tracheal rings
30. ventral
31. vertebrae
32. vestibular fold
33. vocal fold

70. The cranial cavity of the neonate. The skull has been flattened slightly in handling.

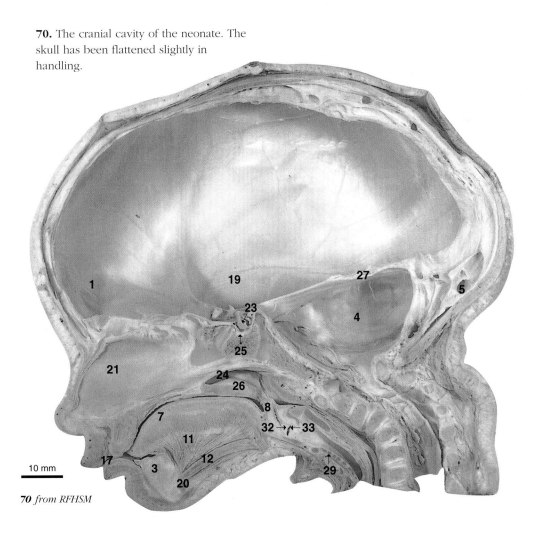

1
19
27
5
23
4
25
21
24
26
8
7
32 33
11
17
12
29
3
20

10 mm

70 *from RFHSM*

71a–71g. Development of the choroid plexus from Day 34 to Week 9.

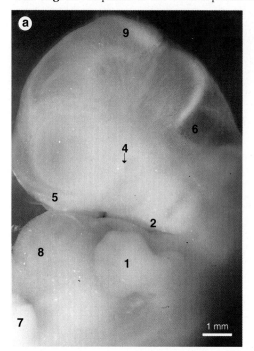

71a. Stage 17 (Day 41). The hindbrain region. 12 mm CR

MENINGES

The meninges are formed when the mesoderm surrounding the neural tube condenses to form the primitive meninx. Dura mater forms from the outer layer of the primitive meninx, and the inner layer (pia-arachnoid), which has neural crest contributions, remains thin. These layers are called the leptomeninges and fluid-filled spaces appearing within this layer coalesce and so form the subarachnoid space. In Week 5 embryonic cerebrospinal fluid begins to form.

CHOROID PLEXUS

Pia mater and blood vessels invaginate the thin inner wall of the hemispheres and the thin thalamic and hindbrain grooves to form the choroid plexus of the lateral, third, and fourth ventricles. These plexuses contribute to cerebrospinal fluid formation.

71b and **71c.** Stage 19 (Days 47–48).

71b. The hindbrain region and the developing choroid plexus of the fourth ventricle. 20 mm CR

71c. A higher magnification of **71b**. The hindbrain roof has been removed.

1. arm bud
2. branchial arch
3. choroid plexus
4. eye
5. forebrain
6. hindbrain
7. leg bud
8. liver bulge
9. midbrain

71d and **71e.** The developing choroid plexus of the cerebral vesicles.

71d. Week 8. 34 mm CR   **71e.** Week 10. 57 mm CR ♂

1. choroid plexus
2. corpus striatum
3. forebrain
4. hindbrain
5. lateral lobe of cerebellum
6. midbrain
7. spinal cord

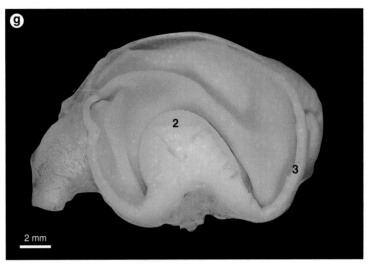

| 1. choroid plexus |
| 2. corpus striatum |
| 3. forebrain |

71f. Week 9. Further development of the choroid plexus of the cerebral vesicles. 48 mm CR ♂

71g. Week 9. Choroid plexus removed from specimen in **71f.**

71h and **71i.** The choroid plexus of the lateral ventricle.

| 1. choroid plexus |
| 2. falx cerebri |
| 3. lateral ventricle |

71h. Week 8. A coronal section of the choroid plexus. 40 mm CR

71b *from St T*

71i. Week 20. Ultrasound scan of the choroid plexus.

| 1. choroid plexus |

71i *from Mr P. Baines*

72a. Stages 16–18 (Days 37–44). Neurohypophysis in sagittal section. 14 mm CR

1. anterior cranial fossa
2. cactus needle
3. cerebellar fossa
4. epiglottis
5. hard palate
6. laryngopharynx
7. mandible
8. mandibular prominence
9. maxilla
10. middle cranial fossa
11. nasal conchae
12. nasopharynx
13. neurohypophysis
14. nose
15. oropharynx
16. pharynx
17. pituitary gland
18. Rathke's pouch
19. sella turcica
20. soft palate
21. tongue
22. vertebral column

Pituitary gland (hypophysis cerebri)

The pituitary gland has dual origins: one part, the adenohypophysis, is an out-pouching of the ectodermal stomodeum (Rathke's pouch) and the other part is a diverticulum of the neuroectodermal diencephalon, called the neurohypophysis. As the pouch tissue enlarges its connection with the mouth eventually atrophies (Week 9). Rathke's pouch forms the *pars distalis*, *pars tuberalis*, and *pars intermedia*. The neurohypophysis and its cavity form the *pars nervosa*, the infundibular stem, and median eminence.

During Weeks 9–17 the pituitary assumes its characteristic shape and histology.

At Weeks 13–14, gonadotrophins are produced by the fetal pituitary. By Weeks 19–20 growth hormone is present.

72b. Week 8. A sagittal section of the pituitary gland and fossa. 37 mm CR

72b from QUB

72c. Week 13. The pituitary gland in the sella turcica. 95 mm CR ♂

72d. The neonatal pituitary gland.

72d from RCS

Eye

FACIAL DEVELOPMENT

One eye forms on each side of the head. They then move medially (Weeks 5–8) on to the front of the face so allowing for binocular vision in later life.

EYE FORMATION

The optic sulci appear on the neural folds in Week 4, and with neural fold fusion form the optic vesicles.

The optic vesicles are two lateral outgrowths of the forebrain (prosencephalic), with lumina at first continuous with the forebrain lumen. The proximal part constricts to form the optic stalk, while the distal portions (optic vesicle) form the retina, part of the iris, and ciliary body. The optic vesicle induces a lens placode in the head ectoderm and indents to form the optic cup. This indentation continues on to the inferior aspect of the optic stalk (optic fetal or choroidal fissure). The two layers of the optic cup appose and together form the retina. As these changes occur the lens placode sinks beneath the ectoderm, detaches, and forms a hollow vesicle.

Vascular mesoderm enters the choroidal fissure and blood vessels grow from the proximal to the distal parts of the optic cup. In Week 7 the fetal fissure fuses and the blood vessels are incorporated into the optic stalk. These vessels form the hyaloid artery and vein which pass from the fissure to the lens. Distally, they degenerate and disappear after Week 31; proximally, they persist as the central artery and vein of the retina.

LENS

The lens begins as a hollow vesicle in which the posterior wall cells hypertrophy and eventually obliterate the cavity. The anterior wall cells persist as a cuboidal anterior lens epithelium. The hypertrophied cells form lens fibers. New lens fibers are added to the mature lens by the equatorial zone cells. The lens capsule is produced by the underlying epithelial cells.

RETINA

The retina forms from the two apposed layers of the optic cup. The outer layer forms the pigmented layer of the retina; the inner layer forms the neural retina. These two layers fuse, but not firmly. Differentiation is confined to the cells in the caudal part of the cup (*pars optica*), which form three zones: ependymal, mantle, and marginal.

The ependymal zone gives rise to the mantle neuroblasts which form two layers: an outer, which forms the bipolar cell layer and possibly the rods and cones, and an inner, which forms the ganglion cells that give rise to the optic nerve. The optic nerve cell axons converge on to the future optic disc region, then change direction to grow centripetally in the marginal zone of the optic stalk. Eventually the stalk lumen disappears. Spongioblasts of the cup give rise to the retinal neuroglia (Muller's fibers).

The inner margin of the optic cup does not differentiate in this manner. The inner layer remains single and, together with the single cell layer of the outer cup, forms first the *pars caeca retinae*, and later the adult *pars iridica retinae*, and the *pars ciliaris retinae*, the posterior epithelial components of the iris and ciliary body.

CHOROID, SCLERA, AND CORNEA

Mesoderm surrounding the optic cup gives rise to the choroid and dura mater of the optic nerve, the sclera, and the *substantia propria corneae*. The stratified squamous corneal epithelium forms from surface ectoderm.

IRIS

Mesoderm immediately anterior to the developing lens gives rise to the pupillary membrane, whose peripheral part together with the *pars iridica retinae* form the iris. The dilator and sphincter pupillae muscles differentiate *in situ*. The center of the pupillary membrane degenerates to form the pupil.

The anterior chamber forms in the mesoderm between the lens and *substantia propria* of the cornea. The posterior chamber is an extension of the anterior chamber.

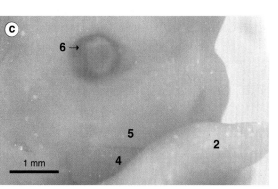

| 1. brain |
| 2. hand |
| 3. lens |
| 4. mandible |
| 5. maxilla |
| 6. pigment |

73a–73i. Development of the eyelids from Day 37 to Week 15.

73a. Stages 16–17 (Days 37–41). Viewed from the side. 12 mm CR

73b. Stages 17–18 (Days 41–44). Viewed from the side. 14 mm CR

73c. Stage 19 (Days 47–48). Viewed from the side. 20 mm CR

LACRIMAL GLANDS

Ectodermal buds from the surface ectoderm branch, canalize, and form the ducts and alveoli during Week 8. The glands are small in the neonate, but function by Week 6. Tears are not produced when the neonate cries.

NASOLACRIMAL DUCT

The nasolacrimal duct forms from an ectodermal cord along a line where the lateral nasal prominence and maxillary prominence meet. The cord later canalizes.

EYELIDS

The eyelids are mesodermal folds covered with ectoderm, which first appear above and below the lens placode and grow toward each other. They fuse at Weeks 9–10 and remain fused until Weeks 25–26. The mesodermal fold gives rise to the tarsal plate and connective tissue; the ectodermal covering gives rise to the tarsal glands and eyelashes.

- Myelination of the optic nerve occurs mainly in the first 3 weeks after birth.
- Slow eye movements occur at Week 14, rapid eye movements at Week 21, and the blink–startle responses at Weeks 22–23.
- In Week 30, the pupillary light reflex can be elicited.

73d. Stage 22 (Day 54). Viewed from the side. 25 mm CR

73e. Stage 22 (Day 54). Viewed from the side. 27 mm CR

73f. Stage 22 (Day 54). Viewed from the side and front. 27 mm CR

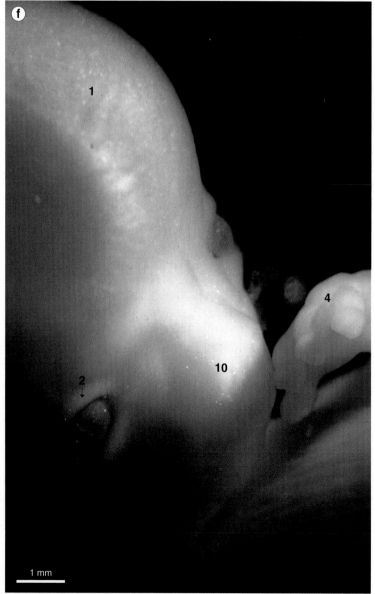

73g. Week 9. Viewed from the front. 46 mm CR

73h. Week 9. Viewed from the front. 48 mm CR

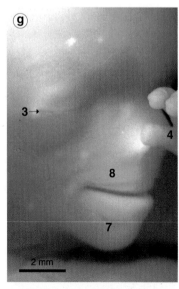

73i. Week 15. Viewed from the front. 130 mm CR ♀

1. brain	**3.** fused eyelids	**5.** lateral angle (outer canthus)	**7.** mandible	**9.** medial angle (inner canthus)	**11.** pigment
2. eyelid	**4.** hand	**6.** lens	**8.** maxilla	**10.** nose	

74a–74f. Coronal sections of the developing eye from Stages 15–16 (Days 33–37) to Week 8.

74a. Stages 15–16 (Days 33–37). 10 mm CR

1. anterior chamber
2. anterior lens cells
3. anterior lens epithelium
4. choroid
5. conjunctival sac
6. cornea
7. corneal ectoderm
8. corneal mesoderm
9. fetal fissure
10. fused eyelids
11. hyaloid artery
12. inferior rectus muscle
13. intraretinal space
14. lens
15. lens fiber
16. lower eyelid
17. nuclei
18. optic cup
19. optic cup: inner layer
20. optic cup: outer layer
21. orbicularis oculi muscle
22. pigmented layer of retina
23. posterior lens cells
24. pupillary membrane
25. sclera
26. upper eyelid
27. vitreous

74e. Stage 23 (Days 56–57). The width of the intraretinal space is exaggerated. 30 mm CR

74a–74f from CCHMS

74b. Stages 16–17 (Days 37–41). 12 mm CR

74c. Stages 16–17 (Days 37–41). The other eye to that in **74b**. 12 mm CR

74f. Week 8. The eyelids have fused. 40 mm CR

74g. Week 8. The lens. 40 mm CR

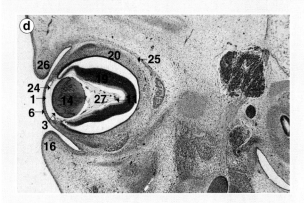

74d. Stage 22 (Day 54). 25 mm CR

74g from St T

Spinal cord

The walls of the neural tube are composed of neuroepithelium which forms three regions: an inner ventricular (ependymal) zone, an intermediate (mantle) zone, and an outer marginal zone. The ventricular layer gives rise to all the spinal cord neurons and macroglial cells. These pass into the intermediate layer and differentiate into neuroblasts and supporting cells so forming the gray matter. The intermediate layer sends axons into the outer marginal zone, which forms the white matter of the cord and contains no cell bodies, only afferent and efferent nerve fibers.

The neuroepithelial cells initially produce neuroblasts, then glioblasts, and finally differentiate into ependymal cells.

As the neuroepithelial cells proliferate and differentiate, the lateral walls of the neural tube thicken until the spinal cord has thin roof and floor plates and a small central canal. Each lateral wall is divided by the *sulcus limitans* into two halves, the dorsal alar and ventral basal plate (lamina). The alar plate with the neural crest will form the sensory apparatus (dorsal or posterior horn) and its associated structures, while the basal plate will form the motor apparatus (ventral or anterior horn). The two sides of the cord are separated by the dorsal septum and the ventral median fissure and septum.

Microglial cells are said to form from mesoderm surrounding the neural tube or possibly from circulating monocytes in the fetal period.

SPINAL NERVES: DORSAL ROOT

Dorsal root ganglia, containing the primary sensory neurons, form from segmental aggregations of neural crest cells. The dorsal root itself consists of processes from these cells extending peripherally (towards sensory receptors) and centrally into the dorsal horn.

SPINAL NERVES: VENTRAL ROOT

Cell axons grow out from the ventral (anterior) horn of gray matter to each somite.

TRACTS

The marginal layer becomes thickened by the development of longitudinally running bundles of nerve fibers (tracts). The first to form are short intersegmental tracts (fasciculi proprii), later followed by the major ascending and descending pathways that connect the spinal cord with the brain.

SPINAL CORD LEVELS

In the embryo, the spinal cord and its associated nerves are present throughout the length of the embryo at Week 8. As the spinal cord grows more slowly than the dura mater and vertebral column, the caudal end of the cord comes to lie at higher vertebral levels. By Week 24 the tip of the cord lies at S1, while in the neonate it is at L3. As these levels are reached, the spinal nerves run obliquely towards the intervertebral foramina to leave the vertebral column. The dura mater extends the length of the

vertebral column, while the pia mater forms the *filum terminale* as the cord retreats.

Myelination begins at about Weeks 17–20 and continues until the age of 1 year.

- In the adult, the spinal cord ends at the lower border of L1. The changes in level should be considered when performing a lumbar puncture on a child.

1. dorsal body wall
2. lamina of vertebra
3. spinal cord
4. vertebral body

75a. Week 13. Sagittal (longitudinal) section of the thoracic spinal cord. 95 mm CR ♂

75b. Week 11. Transverse section of developing lower sacral spinal cord. 65 mm CR

75b from CCHMS

75c. Week 24. The spinal cord no longer occupies the total length of the canal. Exposed from behind.

1. central canal
2. centrum
3. cervical enlargement
4. dorsal horn
5. dorsal nerve root
6. dorsal root ganglion
7. dorsal septum
8. ependymal layer
9. head
10. lumbar enlargement
11. marginal zone
12. neural arch
13. ribs
14. spinal cord
15. spinal nerve
16. ventral horn
17. ventral median fissure

75c from RFHSM

Peripheral nervous system

During Week 5 peripheral nerves grow into the upper and lower limb buds and into the trunk. Dermatomes, or areas of skin supplied by a single spinal nerve and its dorsal root ganglion, are distributed in segmental bands to supply both dorsal and ventral limb surfaces. These patterns are altered as the limbs grow and rotate, but remain relatively unaltered in the trunk.

Autonomic ganglion cells arise from the neural crest. In the case of the sympathetic system, the ganglion cells pass through an intermediate stage in the spinal ganglia and then migrate ventrally. Some come to lie alongside the aorta forming the ganglia of the sympathetic trunk. Initially, this exists only in the thoracic and upper lumbar regions, but later extends cranially and caudally. Some neural crest cells migrate more extensively and form collateral ganglia, such as the celiac and superior mesenteric, and the chromaffin cells of the suprarenal medulla.

The parasympathetic (craniosacral) ganglia are derived from neural crest in the appropriate regions, along with sensory cranial nerve ganglia, such as the trigeminal and facial ganglia.

76. Week 18. Segmental spinal nerves supplying the body wall, view of the left side. 150 mm CR ♀

1. abdomen
2. back
3. elbow
4. latissimus dorsi muscle (position)
5. leg (left)
6. segmental spinal nerves
7. serratus anterior muscle (position)

77a and **77b.** Week 10. The thoracic sympathetic trunk, viewed from the left side. The left lung has been removed.

77a. 56 mm CR

77b. 56 mm CR

1. auricle of heart
2. diaphragm
3. intercostal vessels
4. left superior intercostal vein
5. pericardium (reflected)
6. rami communicantes
7. sympathetic trunk
8. ventricle of heart

Face development

78a–78l. Development of the face from Day 37 to Week 18.

78a. Stages 16–18 (Days 37–44). 14 mm CR

78b. Stages 16–18 (Days 37–44). 14 mm CR

The face develops over a period of time. Initially, the eyes are on the sides of the head, the nostrils are widely separated, the nose flattened, and the ears on the side of the neck.

The face forms as a result of changes in relative position and proportion of five growth centers or primordia: two maxillary and two mandibular prominences and a single median frontonasal prominence. The eyes move medially on the face, the nostrils move medially, and the ears rise on to the head (see Face profile).

78c. Stage 19 (Days 47–48). 20 mm CR

1. arm
2. eye
3. frontonasal process
4. hand
5. leg
6. mandibular prominence
7. maxillary prominence
8. nasal pit
9. nostril
10. thorax
11. umbilical cord

78d. Stage 19 (Days 47–48). 20 mm CR

78e. Stage 22 (Day 54). 27 mm CR

78f. A further view of the face in **78e**.

1. arm
2. eye
3. lips
4. mandible
5. maxilla
6. nose
7. nostril
8. thorax

78g. Week 8. 32 mm CR

78h. Week 9. 48 mm CR ♀

78i. Week 10. 53 mm CR ♂

78j. Week 12. 85 mm CR ♂

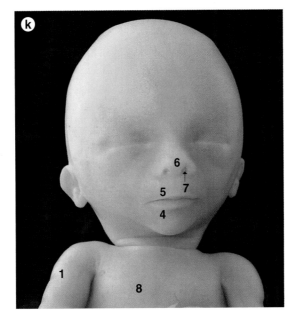

78k. Week 18. 155 mm CR ♀

78l. Week 18. 160 mm CR ♀

Nose

At Week 5 the embryo's eyes are on either side of the head. The nasal placodes are well separated on the front of the face (fronto-nasal prominence) and sinking into the underlying mesoderm to form the nasal pits. The pits are partly on the face and partly in the stomodeum.

The pits or nostrils are blind nasal sacs directed dorsally.

During Weeks 5–6 the nostrils move toward one another and are separated from the oral cavity by the oronasal membrane. The medial nasal prominences fuse with one another to form the intermaxillary segment, which gives rise to the philtrum of the lip, middle portion of the upper jaw, and primary palate. The medial nasal prominences also merge with the maxillary prominences, which are merged with the lateral prominences. The frontonasal process forms the forehead, and bridge and apex of the adult nose, and the lateral nasal prominences form the alae of the adult nose. Ectoderm in the floor of the nasolacrimal groove between the lateral nasal prominence and maxillary prominences forms the nasolacrimal duct.

The blind end of the nostril grows rapidly inward on either side of the midline. The oronasal membrane breaks down and connects the blind tubes of the nostrils (the nasal cavity) with the nasopharynx. The openings are called the primitive choanae (naris). The nasal septum forms from the medial nasal prominences and it is in contact with the dorsum of the tongue.

Projections of the lateral walls form the inferior, middle, and superior conchae. The ectodermal roof of each nasal cavity forms the olfactory region, some of which cells form olfactory cells whose nerve fibers grow into the olfactory bulb through the cribriform plate of the ethmoid bone.

- If fusion is incomplete (hare lip) the maxillary division of the trigeminal nerve is unable to spread to the philtrum of the lip. Instead, the ophthalmic division enters the philtrum from above.
- The neonate breathes primarily through the nose and will only breathe through the mouth when nasal obstruction produces stress.

79a–79n. Development of the nose from a nasal pit to nostril.

79a. Stages 16–18 (Days 37–44). The nasal pits are widely separated on the developing face, viewed from the right side and front. 14 mm CR

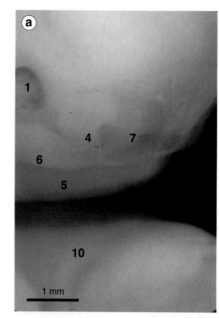

1. eye
2. forehead
3. frontonasal process
4. lateral nasal prominence (alar process)
5. mandibular prominence
6. maxillary prominence
7. medial nasal prominence
8. nasal pit
9. stomodeum
10. thorax

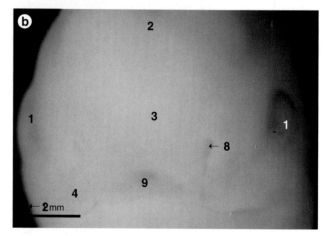

79b. The same embryo as in **79a**, viewed from the front of the face.

1. lateral nasal prominence (alar process)
2. heart
3. medial nasal prominence
4. nostril
5. nasal pit

79c. Stages 15–16 (Days 33–37). Transverse paraffin wax section through the developing nasal pit which ends as a blind sac. 10 mm CR

79d. Section posterior to that shown in **79c**.

79e. Stage 19 (Days 47–48). Embryo viewed from the front of the face. The eyes and nostrils are still widely separated, but have moved toward the front and midline of the face. 20 mm CR

79f. Higher magnification of the embryo in **79e.**

79g and **79h.** The roof of the stomodeum (oral cavity) of the embryo shown in **79e.**

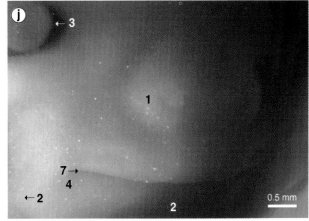

79i. Stage 22 (Day 54). The developing nostril in profile. Note the plugged nostril. 27 mm CR

79j. Same embryo as in **79i**, viewed from the front and right side.

1. alae
2. chin
3. eye
4. forebrain
5. hand
6. maxillary prominence
7. mouth
8. nostril
9. posterior choana (naris)

79k. Week 9. Viewed from the front. The nostrils are widely separated and directed forward. 46 mm CR

79l. Week 10. Viewed from the front. 53 mm CR ♂

79m. Week 10. Viewed from below. 60 mm CR ♀

79n. Week 15. The nostrils are pointed downward. 130 mm CR ♀

1. bridge of the nose
2. chin
3. eye
4. forehead
5. lanugo hair
6. lip
7. nose
8. nostril
9. palate
10. philtrum of the lip
11. plug in the nostril

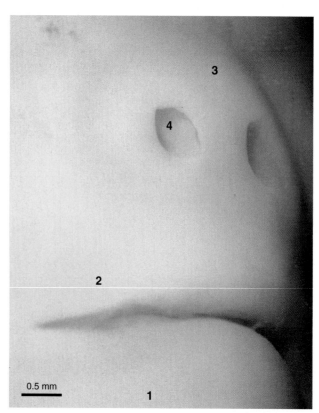

80. Week 9. Fetus with the plugs washed from the developing nostril. 41 mm CR

1. mandible
2. maxilla
3. nose
4. nostril

81. Week 13. The normal sensory distribution of the trigeminal nerve on the face. 92 mm CR ♀

1. maxillary division
2. mandibular division
3. ophthalmic division

82. Week 18. A hemisection (sagittal) of the head. The black thread through the nostril marks the extent of the nasopharynx.

82 from RCS

1. cranial fossa (middle)
2. diaphragm
3. heart
4. mandible
5. nose
6. nasopharynx
7. spinal cord
8. sternum
9. thymus
10. tongue
11. vertebrae

83a–83l. The developing profile of the face.

83a. Stages 17 (Day 41). 12 mm CR

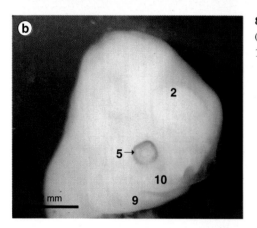

83b. Stages 16–18 (Days 37–44). 14 mm CR

83c. Stage 19 (Days 47–48). 20 mm CR

Face profile

The profile changes dramatically; originally, the forehead dominates the face (Stages 16–17, Days 37–41) and the mandible is more advanced in development than the maxilla. The nose and maxilla then grow rapidly (Stage 19, Days 47–48) and, in the early fetal period, the mandible lags behind so the embryo lacks a well-developed chin and its face has a simian appearance.

During Weeks 8–12 the mandible grows rapidly, and the deep indentation between the nose and forehead is lost as the bridge of the nose is elevated. The nostrils, which were widely separated and directed forward, are then pointed downward.

1. arm
2. brain
3. bridge of the nose
4. ear
5. eye
6. hand
7. leg
8. lips
9. mandible
10. maxilla
11. nose
12. nostril

83d. Week 8. 35 mm CR

83e. Week 9. 43 mm CR

83f. Week 9. 45 mm CR

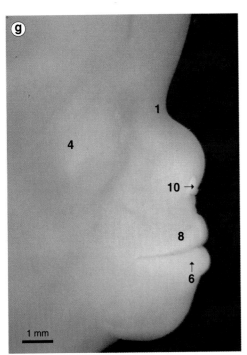

83g. Week 9. 48 mm CR ♀

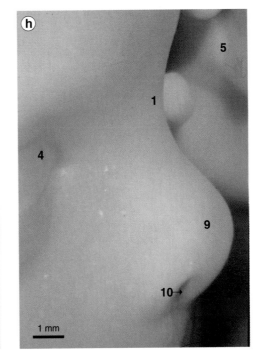

83h. Week 12. 85 mm CR ♂

1. bridge of the nose
2. brain
3. ear
4. eye
5. hand
6. lips
7. mandible
8. maxilla
9. nose
10. nostril

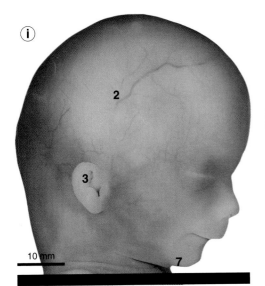

83i. Week 13. 92 mm CR ♀

83j. Week 18. 160 mm CR ♀

83k. Week 24. 228 mm CR ♂

83l from RCS

83l. The profile of the neonate.

Mandible and maxilla

The first branchial arch on each side of the head divides into two processes: maxillary and mandibular prominences which grow toward the midline. The two mandibular prominences (processes) fuse first (Week 4) and the maxillary processes fuse with the frontonasal process in Weeks 6–7. The outer corners of the mouth are defined by Week 5 and this broad mouth opening is later reduced during the first half of Week 6 by the lips fusing laterally at the corners. The cheeks then form. The labial and buccal muscles form from the second branchial arch mesoderm.

Meckel's cartilage forms from the first arch and serves as 'scaffolding' for the membrane bone of the mandible. Neural crest cells in the arches form the skeletal and connective tissue of the lower face and anterior neck.

The primitive mouth is an ectoderm-lined depression (stomodeum) separated from the foregut by the oropharyngeal (buccopharyngeal) membrane. In Week 4 the oral membrane ruptures and the foregut communicates with the amniotic cavity.

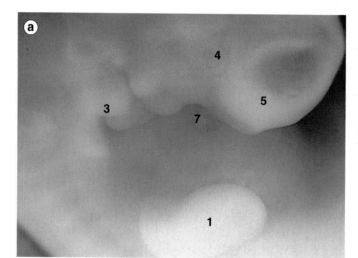

84a–84g. Development of the mandible and maxilla. The mandible and maxilla are represented by two arch prominences from the first branchial arch.

84a. Stage 16 (Day 37). View from the right side. 12 mm CR

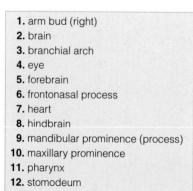

1. arm bud (right)
2. brain
3. branchial arch
4. eye
5. forebrain
6. frontonasal process
7. heart
8. hindbrain
9. mandibular prominence (process)
10. maxillary prominence
11. pharynx
12. stomodeum

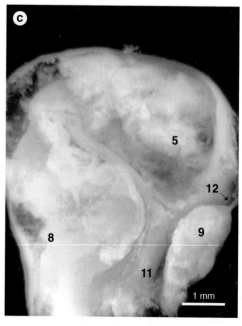

84b. Stages 16–18 (Days 37–44). View from the front. 14 mm CR

84c. Stages 16–18 (Days 37–44). A hemisection of the head, view from the medial surface. 14 mm CR

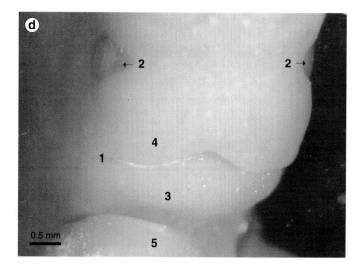

84d. Stage 19 (Days 47–48). View from the front. The maxillary prominences (processes) and medial nasal prominences have fused to form the maxilla. Note the wide mouth and the eyes still placed on either side of the head. 20 mm CR

1. angle of mouth
2. eye
3. mandibular prominence
4. maxillary prominence
5. thorax

84e. Stage 22 (Day 54). View from the right side. Note the angles of the mouth are fusing to form a less broad mouth. 27 mm CR

84f. Week 9. View from the right and front of the fetus. Note the eyes and nose are not yet in their final positions on the face. 43 mm CR

1. angle of mouth
2. arm
3. chin
4. eye
5. hand
6. lip
7. mandible
8. maxilla
9. nose
10. ribs

84g. Week 8. The skin has been removed from the mandible to illustrate the developing bone, viewed from the right side. 40 mm CR

Lips and teeth

The early mouth is bounded by the fused mandibular prominences and the fused maxillary and medial nasal prominences. These boundaries divide (Weeks 6–10) into the lips (labia) and gums (gingiva). In Week 6 an ectodermal thickening, the dental lamina, grows into the underlying mesoderm. A second ectodermal thickening, the labiogingival lamina, grows into the mesoderm between the dental lamina and the future lip.

As the teeth develop the labiogingival lamina degenerates and leaves a groove which deepens and separates the lips, cheeks, and gums. One small area does not completely degenerate and forms the midline lingual frenulum, attaching the upper lip to the gingiva.

The dental laminae in each jaw form ten oval buds, which will form the enamel organ primordia of the deciduous teeth (milk teeth). These are followed at Week 10 by the first permanent teeth buds which form lingual to the deciduous teeth. The laminae then disappear.

Based on their appearance the tooth buds progress through a cap stage and finally a bell stage.

Early in Week 7 the mesoderm deep to the enamel organ condenses to form a dental papilla (cap stage). The dental papilla will give rise to the dentin and pulp.

In the bell stage, the dental papilla mesoderm differentiates into dentin-forming odontoblasts. The earliest dentin formed is

85a and **85b.** Week 8. Coronal sections of cap stages of tooth development.

85a. 32 mm CR

85b. 40 mm CR

85c–85g. Coronal sections of tooth development in the mandible (bell stage).

85c. Week 8. 36 mm CR

1. ameloblast layer	**7.** intermediate layer	**13.** outer epithelium
2. dental ledge	**8.** labiogingival lamina	**14.** palate
3. dentin	**9.** mandible	**15.** pulp
4. developing muscle	**10.** mesodermal pulp	**16.** stellate reticulum
5. enamel	primordium (dental papilla)	**17.** tongue
6. enamel organ of milk teeth	**11.** odontoblast layer	
(deciduous teeth)	**12.** oral epithelium	

85d. Week 13. 100 mm CR

85f and **85g.** Week 28. 270 mm CR.

85e. Week 14. 120 mm CR

85d and 85e from CCHMS 85c, 85f, and 85g from QUB

the outermost layer formed until the papilla is reduced and the remaining mesoderm cells form the pulp. Odontoblast processes remaining in the dentin are called Tomes' odontoblastic fibers. Mesoderm surrounding the enamel organ and dental papilla condenses to form the dental sac, which will form cementum and the periodontal ligament. By Week 14 cells of the inner part of the enamel organ differentiate into ameloblasts and form enamel, the deepest layer being the first to be laid down. Enamel is laid down at the cusp first and progresses toward the root, as does dentin formation. The root is formed as the enamel epithelium (epithe-lial root sheath) grows into adjacent mesoderm. Odontoblasts adjacent to the sheath form dentin continuous with the crown.

- Permanent molars with no deciduous predecessors develop as buds from the dental laminae.
- The teeth do not all develop at the same time.
- The root of the tooth forms shortly before eruption.
- The neonatal jaw contains the completed crowns of the 20 deciduous teeth and the primordia of all the 32 permanent teeth except the second and third molars.

86a. Stage 19 (Days 47–48). View from the right side. 20 mm CR

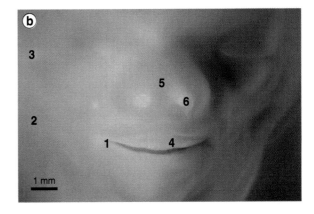

86b. Week 9. View from the front. 46 mm CR

86a–86c. Development of the lips.

1. angle of the mouth
2. cheek
3. eye
4. lip
5. nose
6. nostril with plug

86c. Week 18. 160 mm CR ♂

86d and **86e.** Week 8. Sagittal section through the lips, palate, and tongue. 36 mm CR

86e. Lip.

1. esophagus
2. lip
3. hard palate
4. hypophysis
5. nose
6. oral epithelium
7. skin
8. soft palate
9. tongue

86d and *86e* *from QUB*

Palate

Three palatal processes develop and will separate the nasal cavity and the mouth: the primary palate (or median palatine process) and the secondary palate (two lateral palatine processes). The primary and secondary palate form between Weeks 5–12. The primary palate forms in Week 6 from the fusion of the two medial nasal prominences (see Nose). The secondary palate forms when the dorsum of the tongue, which is pressed against the nasal septum (Week 7), withdraws. The two lateral palatine processes, which originally projected vertically downward on either side of the tongue, meet in the midline and fuse. They also fuse with the primary palate and nasal septum and together form an horizontal shelf. Fusion occurs between Weeks 7–12.

Membrane bone in the primary palate forms the premaxilla; while bone from the maxillae and the palatine bones extend into the lateral palatine processes to form the hard palate. The soft palate and uvula extend beyond the nasal septum and do not become ossified.

- If the processes fail to fuse, the nasal cavity and mouth remain in continuity. This condition, known as cleft palate, interferes with feeding and speech.
- The neonatal hard palate is short and broad, while the adult palate is deeply arched.

87a and **87b.** Stage 19 (Days 47–48). The palate, two views of the same embryo. 20 mm CR

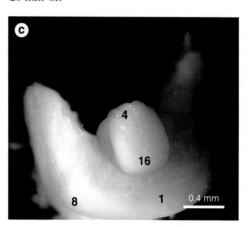

87c. The mandible and tongue of the embryo in **87a**. The tongue is positioned in a groove on the mandibular process.

1. chin	
2. developing gum	
3. developing lip	
4. dorsum of the tongue	
5. eye	
6. forehead	
7. lateral palatine process	
8. mandible	
9. maxilla	
10. maxillary process	
11. nasal septum	
12. nostril	
13. palatine raphe	
14. primary palate	
15. secondary palate	
16. tip of the tongue	
17. uvula	

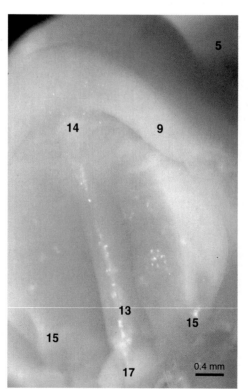

88. Week 8. The two lateral palatine processes and median palatine process have fused in the mid-line. The uvula remains unfused. 35 mm CR

89a. Week 9. The frenulum and gums of the maxilla are beginning to be distinguishable. The mandible has been removed. 48 mm CR ♂

1. eye
2. frenulum
3. gum
4. lip
5. maxilla
6. nose

89b. Week 11. The uvula has fused in the mid-line. 65 mm CR ♂

1. eye
2. frenulum
3. gum
4. hard palate
5. lip
6. maxilla
7. nasopharynx
8. nostril
9. palatine raphe
10. philtrum of the lip
11. soft palate
12. uvula

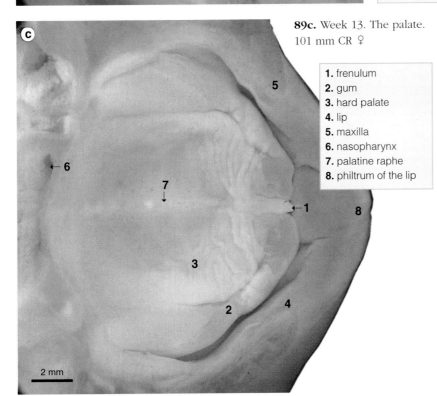

89c. Week 13. The palate. 101 mm CR ♀

1. frenulum
2. gum
3. hard palate
4. lip
5. maxilla
6. nasopharynx
7. palatine raphe
8. philtrum of the lip

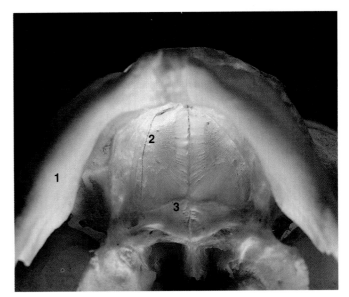

90. The neonatal bony palate, viewed from below.

1. mandible
2. maxilla
3. maxillary process of the palatine bone

91a and **91b.** The unfused and fused palate in transverse paraffin wax sections.

1. arytenoid swelling
2. cartilaginous otic capsule
3. Eustachian tube
4. fused lateral palatine processes
5. hindbrain (medulla)
6. hyoid cartilage
7. lateral palatine processes
8. maxilla
9. Meckel's cartilage
10. nasal cavity
11. nasal septum
12. oral cavity
13. semicircular canals
14. submandibular gland
15. thyroid cartilage
16. tongue
17. tooth

91a. Stage 21 (Day 52). 24 mm CR

91b. Week 8. 32 mm CR

91a and 91b from CCHMS

92. Week 17. The fused palate in a sagittal (longitudinal) section. 150 mm CR

1. aorta
2. atrium of heart
3. cerebellum
4. diaphragm
5. ductus venosus
6. esophagus
7. feet
8. fingers
9. hard palate
10. intestines
11. lip
12. liver
13. lung
14. nasal cavity
15. nose
16. phallus
17. pituitary
18. soft palate
19. sternum
20. urinary bladder
21. ventricle of heart
22. vertebrae

5 mm

92 from CCHMS

Tongue

The anterior two-thirds of the tongue (body) forms during Week 4 from the fusion of a median swelling (median tongue bud, *tuberculum impar*) in the floor of the pharynx between the first pair of branchial arches and the two distal tongue buds (lateral lingual swellings) derived from each first arch. The two distal buds overgrow and bury the median bud as they grow medially. The median sulcus marks the fusion of the two distal buds.

The posterior third of the tongue (root) forms from the fusion of the ventromedial ends of the second arches to form the copula. A large hypobranchial eminence develops caudal to the copula from third and fourth arch mesoderm. This eminence overgrows the copula which disappears.

The boundary between the two areas is the sulcus terminalis, with the thyroid rudiment (the *foramen cecum*) in the midline. The papillae develop at Weeks 7–9 and the taste buds during Weeks 11–13. Most of the muscles develop from occipital myotomes.

- The neonatal tongue is within the oral cavity. The posterior third will descend into the neck after birth (1–5 years) to form part of the anterior pharyngeal wall.

Larynx

The proximal end of the laryngotracheal (respiratory) diverticulum, the larynx, develops from the endodermal lining of the laryngotracheal diverticulum and neural crest cells and surrounding mesoderm (fourth and sixth branchial arches). In Weeks 5 and 6 three swellings appear, one called the epiglottal swelling (from the third and fourth branchial arches) and two arytenoid swellings. Together the three swellings make the opening to the trachea 'Y' or 'T' shaped. Later, the corniculate and arytenoid cartilages form from the arytenoid swellings.

In Weeks 7–10 the laryngeal epithelium fuses and the entrance ends blindly. In Week 10 the larynx recanalizes and two lateral recesses, the laryngeal ventricles, are formed, as well as the vestibular and vocal folds; the laryngeal aditus slowly enlarges.

The laryngeal muscles and cartilages are fourth and sixth branchial arch derivatives.

- Before the posterior third of the tongue descends into the neck (first to fifth years of postnatal development) the opening of the larynx is directly below the oral cavity.
- Owing to its high position in the neck, the neonatal epiglottis can make direct contact with the soft palate, which assists in directing fluid and breathing freely during suckling.

1. arytenoid swellings	**6.** epiglottis
2. brain	**7.** floor of pharynx (one tuberculum
3. buccopharyngeal membrane	impar and two mandibular swellings)
4. developing tongue	**8.** mandibular prominence
5. dorsum of tongue	**9.** red cactus needle

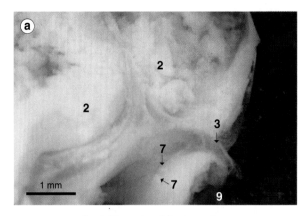

93a. Stages 16–18 (Days 37–44). Sagittal section through the left side of the developing pharynx and brain. 14 mm CR

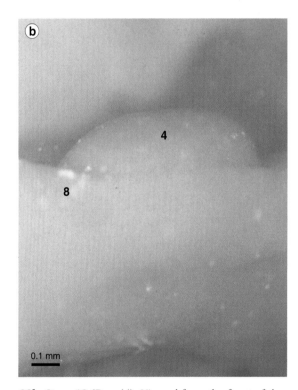

93b. Stage 18 (Day 44). Viewed from the front of the face. 16 mm CR

93c. Stage 19 (Days 47–48). Dorsum of the tongue. 20 mm CR

94a. Week 8. 40 mm CR

1. arytenoid swellings
2. dorsum of tongue
3. epiglottis

94b. Week 8. A transverse section through the larynx. 40 mm CR

1. arytenoid cartilage
2. epiglottis
3. laryngeal aditus

94b from St T

94c. Week 9. 48 mm CR ♂

94d. Week 11. 65 mm CR ♂

1. arytenoid swellings
2. dorsum of tongue
3. epiglottis
4. mandible
5. vallate papillae

95. Week 13. The tongue. 101 mm CR ♀

1. arytenoid swellings
2. epiglottis
3. fungiform papillae
4. lip
5. mandible
6. sulcus terminalis
7. vallate papillae

15 mm

96 from RCS

96. Sagittal section of a neonatal head to illustrate the position of the developed tongue and larynx.

1. cerebellar fossa
2. confluence of sinuses
3. epiglottis
4. genioglossus muscle
5. hard palate
6. lips
7. mandible
8. mylohyoid muscle
9. nasal cavity
10. note the absence of a developed frontal sinus
11. pharynx
12. soft palate
13. tentorium cerebelli

97a. Week 8. Longitudinal section of the developing tongue. 35 mm CR

97a from Mr G. Bottomly

97b. Week 8. Transverse section of the developing tongue. 40 mm CR

97b from St T

1. dental ledge	8. nasal cavity
2. genioglossus muscle	9. inferior longitudinal muscle
3. geniohyoid muscle	10. superior longitudinal muscle
4. hard palate	11. vertical muscle and transverse
5. lip	muscle
6. mandible	(9–11 intrinsic muscles of the
7. maxilla	tongue)

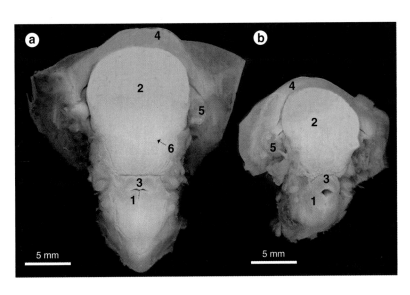

5 mm

5 mm

98a and **98b.** Development of the epiglottis and arytenoid swellings, views of the dorsum of the tongue.

98a. Week 13. 101 mm CR ♀

98b. Week 13. 92 mm CR ♀

1. arytenoid swellings
2. dorsum of the tongue
3. epiglottis
4. lip
5. mandible
6. sulcus terminalis

Salivary glands

The first pair of salivary glands to develop are the parotid glands (Weeks 6–7). The submandibular glands develop late in Week 6 and the sublingual glands at Week 8.

All three pairs of glands develop from solid epithelial outgrowths of the oral cavity which penetrate into the surrounding mesoderm. The tips of the outgrowths form branches and terminal acini. By Weeks 10–12 the solid outgrowths, branches, and acini develop lumens. The main outgrowths form the main ducts of the salivary glands and all the secretory tissue. Neural crest cells give rise to the connective tissue.

The parotid gland outgrowth develops from the ectodermal lining of the mouth, while the submandibular and sublingual glands develop from endodermal outgrowths.

- Secretory activity begins at Week 16 in the submandibular glands and at Week 18 in the parotid glands.
- In the 2 years following birth, all three pairs of salivary glands develop the typical adult histological appearance.
- In the neonate the sublingual gland is continuous with the deep portion of the submandibular gland.
- The parotid gland is round at birth and gradually grows over the surface of the parotid duct in early childhood.

99a–99c. Lateral view of the left parotid gland.

99a. Week 11. 65 mm CR ♂

99b. Week 13. 95 mm CR ♀

99c. Week 18. 152 mm CR ♂

1. branches of the facial nerve
2. buccal fat pad
3. ear
4. eye
5. fat
6. mouth
7. nose
8. orbicularis oculi
9. parotid gland

99d. Week 8. Transverse paraffin wax section through the nasal septum and tongue. 32 mm CR ♂

1. arytenoid swelling
2. developing tooth
3. inferior concha
4. Meckel's cartilage
5. nasal septum
6. palate
7. submandibular gland
8. tongue

Ear: external

AURICLE

A series of six auricular hillocks appears around the first branchial groove, three on each of the first (mandibular) and second (hyoid) arches,

The tubercles on each arch fuse together to form the auricle (pinna) of the ear, only the most ventral on the first arch is recognizable as the tragus. Mesoderm of the hyoid arch proliferates to complete the auricle. The auricles form initially in the neck region, but move up on to the head by Week 10.

EXTERNAL ACOUSTIC MEATUS

The external acoustic (auditory) meatus develops at the dorsal end of the first branchial groove as a funnel-shaped tube (primary meatus). Ectoderm cells at the inner end of the primary meatus proliferate to form a meatal plug. Later this degenerates to form a cavity, the inner part of the external acoustic meatus.

The early tympanic membrane (or eardrum) is the first branchial membrane. Later, mesoderm enters and the tympanic membrane is formed from ectoderm of the first branchial groove, mesoderm from the first and second branchial arches, and tubotympanic recess endoderm.

- The shape of the fully formed auricles varies greatly from individual to individual.
- The tympanic membrane completes its growth by birth.
- The lumen of the neonatal external acoustic meatus is filled with a sebaceous secretion, the *vernix caseosa*, and desquamated epithelial cells.
- At birth the stylomastoid foramen and the emerging facial nerve lie unprotected near the surface, as the mastoid process does not develop until 2 years of age.

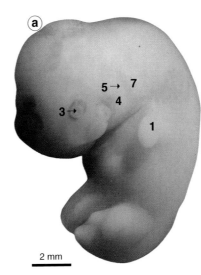

2 mm

100a–100j. Development of the auricle and external acoustic meatus.

1. arm bud
2. external acoustic meatus
3. eye
4. first arch (mandibular)
5. first branchial groove
6. mandible
7. second arch (hyoid)
8. tubercles (hillocks)

100a. Stages 16–17 (Days 37–41). 12 mm CR

100b. Stages 17 (Day 41). 12 mm CR

0.5 mm

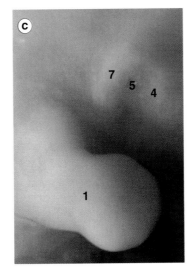

100c. Stage 18 (Day 44). 16 mm CR

0.5 mm

100d. Stage 19 (Days 47–48). 20 mm CR

1. auricle (pinna)
2. tragus

100e. Stage 22 (Day 54). 27 mm CR

100f. Stage 22 (Day 54). 27 mm CR

100g. Week 8. 35 mm CR

100h. Week 9. 48 mm CR ♂

100i. Week 13. 95 mm CR ♂

100j. Week 15. 130 mm CR ♀

100k. Week 24. Origins of the ear. The continuous line encloses the area derived from the first arch, the broken line encloses the area derived from the second arch. 228 mm CR ♂

Ear: internal

The otic placodes are ectodermal thickenings (with a possible contribution of neuroectoderm) on the hindbrain region immediately caudal to the acousticofacial mass which sink below the surface and form otic vesicles (otocysts) (Week 4). The otocysts give rise to the membranous labyrinth of the inner ear.

INNER EAR

A hollow diverticulum, which will form the endolymphatic duct and sac, appears on the upper medial aspect of the otocyst. The upper and lower parts of the otocyst enlarge to form two areas: the utricular (vestibular) and saccular (cochlear) divisions; the constriction between them forms the utriculosaccular duct. Three circular pouches arise from the utricular part and their central walls fuse and are resorbed. Their peripheral walls remain as the semicircular ducts. The lateral canal lies horizontally, the superior canal lies in the frontal plane, the posterior canal lies initially in a frontal plane, and then swings through 90° to lie sagittally. The superior and posterior canals share the *crus commune* into the utricular part of the otocyst.

The saccular part of the otocysts divides into two regions: an upper expanded part which will form the saccule, while the lower coils two and a half times to form the cochlear duct and then the membranous cochlea. The constriction separating the saccule and cochlear duct is the *ductus reuniens.*

The epithelium in six regions modifies to neuroepithelium; a crista in the ampulla of each semicircular duct, two maculae (one each in the utricle and saccule), and the spiral organ (of Corti) along the duct of the cochlea.

The geniculate ganglion of the facial nerve separates from the acousticofacial complex; the remaining complex divides into two regions, the vestibular and cochlear (spiral) ganglia. The vestibular ganglion sends processes to the maculae and cristae, and the spiral organ of Corti receives processes from the cochlear ganglion.

Mesoderm surrounding the otic vesicle forms the cartilaginous otic capsule. Vacuoles appear in the capsule, coalesce, and form the perilymphatic spaces. The enlarging membranous labyrinth is now suspended in perilymph. The bony (osseous) labyrinth of the middle ear is the remaining ossified otic capsule.

- By Weeks 20–22 the inner ear has reached adult size.

MIDDLE EAR

The middle ear forms between the developing internal (inner) ear and the external acoustic meatus.

The tubotympanic recess, which is an endodermal derivative from the first pouch, grows between the otocyst and the external acoustic (auditory) meatus. The distal end of the diverticulum expands to form the tympanic cavity. The proximal part forms the auditory or pharyngotympanic (Eustachian) tube. The developing middle ear cavity surrounds the three ossicles (malleus, incus, and stapes), their muscles, and the *chorda tympani* nerve so that they project into the cavity like a peninsula covered with recess epithelium. The malleus and incus have formed from Meckel's cartilage (first arch) and the stapes from Reichert's cartilage (second arch). The tensor tympani muscle forms from the first arch mesoderm and the stapedius muscle from the second. The muscles are supplied by their arch nerves, the mandibular and facial nerve, respectively.

In the late fetus the tympanic cavity expands and gives rise to the tympanic or mastoid antrum.

- Fetuses prefer rhythmic sound to excessively loud, soft, simple, or complex noises.
- At birth, amniotic fluid and fluid secreted by the respiratory tract are often found in the cavity of the middle ear.
- In the neonate the course of the auditory tube is horizontal and enters the pharynx at the junction of the hard and soft palates. By 5 or 6 years of age the opening has shifted up to lie posterior to the inferior concha.
- The majority of the mastoid air cells form after birth. The mastoid process appears by 2 years of age and grows primarily between the age of 3 years to puberty.
- In the infant and young child, the petrosquamous fissure of the mastoid temporal bone opens directly into the mastoid antrum of the middle ear and is a route for middle ear infection to spread to the meninges.

101. Stage 21 (Day 52). Transverse paraffin wax section of the developing semicircular canals. 24 mm CR

1. cartilaginous otic capsule
2. Eustachian tube
3. hindbrain (medulla)
4. lateral palatine processes
5. semicircular canals
6. tongue

101 from CCHMS

102a. Week 8. 40 mm CR   *102a from St T*

102b. Week 13. 95 mm CR

102c. Week 15. 130 mm CR   *102b and 102c from CCHMS*

102d. Week 21. Horizontal section through the left ear.   *102d from Dr J. Wakely*

102a–102d. Paraffin wax sections of the developing ear.

1. cartilage
2. cochlea
3. cochlear duct
4. first arch derivatives
5. internal auditory meatus
6. internal carotid artery
7. petrous temporal bone
8. trigeminal (V) nerve ganglion
9. vestibule
10. vestibulocochlear (VIII) nerve

103. Neonatal incus and stapes.

2 mm

1. incus
2. stapes

5 mm

104. Weeks 13–14. The head and neck dissected to show elements of the first and second branchial arches.

1. hyoid bone
2. incus
3. malleus
4. mandible
5. Meckel's cartilage
6. stylohyoid ligament
7. tympanic ring

104 from RFHSM

Pharynx

BRANCHIAL OR PHARYNGEAL ARCHES AND GROOVES

Early in Week 4 a series of paired swellings appear on either side of the midline in the future head and neck region. They are present both externally and internally. These branchial arches support the cranial foregut region or pharynx. The foregut extends from the oral membrane to the entry of the bile duct. At the end of Week 4 six pairs of branchial arches are present, the last two being rudimentary. The fifth arch may be absent. Usually only three pairs are apparent externally. Each arch is separated from the next by a branchial groove or cleft. The external appearance is similar to the gills and gill slits in a fish. Of the six arches, the first is also known as the mandibular arch and the second as the hyoid arch. The first arch is divided into two prominences or processes; one forms the mandible, and the second contributes to the maxilla. The second arch contributes to the hyoid bone and the adjacent area. Each arch is covered by ectoderm externally, foregut endoderm internally, and has a core of mesoderm. Neural crest cells, which make a major contribution to head mesoderm, migrate into each arch and surround the arch mesodermal core. The mesoderm and the neural crest will form muscles, skeletal and connective tissues. Each arch also contains an artery, a cartilaginous bar, and a nerve which has grown from the brain.

During Week 5 the hyoid arch overgrows the third and fourth arches to form the cervical sinus. Gradually, the grooves and the cervical sinus become less recognizable and the neck is smooth.

Branchial arch muscles form striated muscles in the head and neck.

The branchial arch nerves are: first – trigeminal, second – facial, third – glossopharyngeal, fourth – superior laryngeal branch of vagus, and sixth – recurrent laryngeal branch of vagus.

For branchial arch artery derivatives, see Blood vessels; and for branchial arch cartilage derivatives, see Skull and arch derivatives.

PHARYNGEAL POUCHES

The foregut endoderm lines the inner aspect of the branchial arches as they bulge into the pharynx. Each arch is separated from the next by a groove or cleft called a pharyngeal pouch. In the pouch, the endoderm contacts the ectoderm of the branchial groove to form the branchial or pharyngeal membrane. The first pouches are clearly defined, while the fifth is rudimentary or absent.

The first dorsal pouch forms the tubotympanic recess (tympanic cavity, mastoid antrum, and the auditory tube); the second dorsal pouch contributes to the palatine tonsil. The ventral parts of the first and second pouches are obliterated by tongue formation. The third dorsal pouch forms the inferior parathyroids, while the ventral third pouch forms the thymus gland. The fourth dorsal pouch gives rise to the superior parathyroids and the fourth ventral pouch to the ultimobranchial body.

105a. Stages 11–12 (Days 23–27). The pharyngeal region. 4 mm CR

105a from CCHMS

1. aortic arch	7. neural crest
2. branchial arch (two)	8. optic vesicle
3. branchial groove	9. pharyngeal pouch
4. dorsal aorta	10. prosencephalon (diencephalon)
5. mandibular prominence (process)	11. stomodeum
6. maxillary prominence (process)	12. thyroid diverticulum

105b. Stage 17 (Day 41). The pharyngeal region. 12 mm CR

1. arm bud (left)
2. branchial arches
3. forebrain
4. heart
5. hindbrain

105c. Stages 14–15 (Days 32–33). Transverse section of the pharyngeal region. 7 mm CR

105c from LHSM

105d. Stages 15–16 (Days 33–37) Sagittal section of the pharyngeal region. 10 mm CR

105d from CCHMS

1. aortic arch (two)	5. hypoglossal nerve (XII)	9. neurohypophysis
2. branchial arch (one)	6. liver	10. optic cup
3. eye	7. myotome	11. otic area
4. heart	8. nasal area	

Neck

By approximately the end of Week 8, the embryo has developed a neck. This is the result of partial extension of the head.

● An important feature of neck development is the associated 'descent' of the heart.
● Extension of the head is important in palate formation during Weeks 8–10.
● At birth, the neck and trunk musculature are not sufficiently developed to support the large head which should be supported when lifting the infant.

106a–106c. Development of the neck.

106a. Stage 16 (Day 37). 12 mm CR

106b. Stage 19 (Days 47–48). 20 mm CR

106c. Week 13. 92 mm CR ♀

| 1. amnion and chorion |
| 2. arm |
| 3. brain |
| 4. heart |
| 5. leg |
| 6. liver |
| 7. neck |
| 8. umbilical cord |

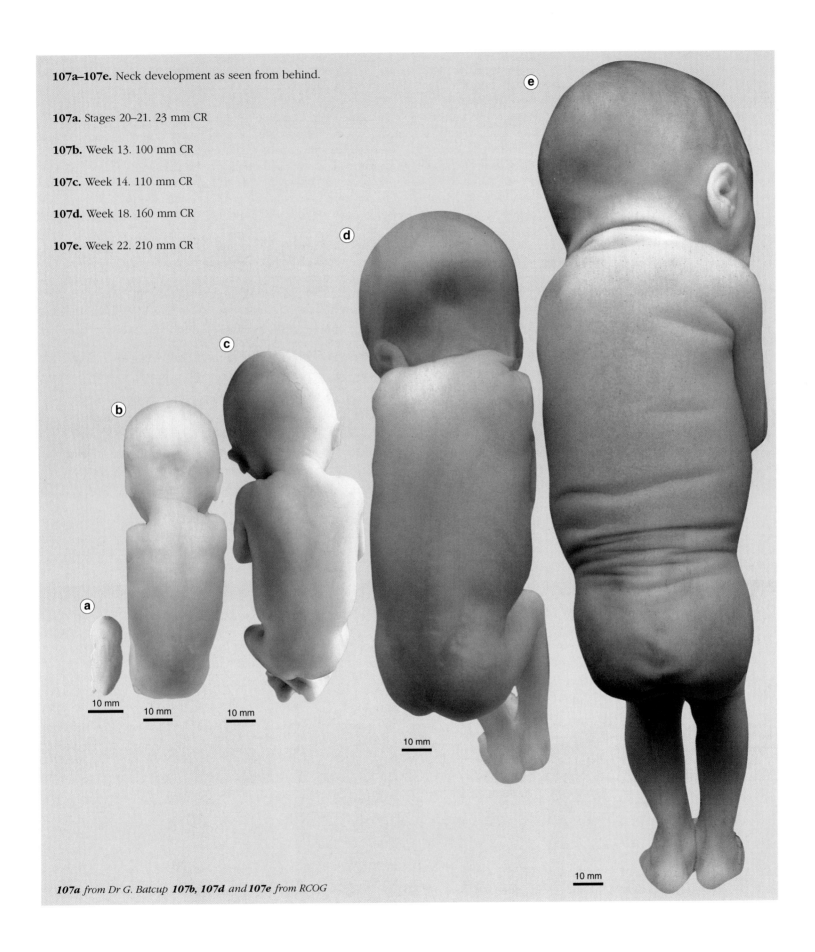

107a–107e. Neck development as seen from behind.

107a. Stages 20–21. 23 mm CR

107b. Week 13. 100 mm CR

107c. Week 14. 110 mm CR

107d. Week 18. 160 mm CR

107e. Week 22. 210 mm CR

10 mm

10 mm

10 mm

10 mm

10 mm

107a *from Dr G. Batcup* **107b, 107d** *and* **107e** *from RCOG*

Thyroid

During Weeks 3–4 a median hollow endodermal thyroid diverticulum appears in the floor of the pharynx opposite the first and second pharyngeal pouches. It forms a bilobed solid diverticulum which is in close contact with the aortic sac and as the sac migrates caudally during neck development, the thyroid migrates to its position in the neck. During migration the gland passes ventral to the hyoid bone and laryngeal cartilages, its stalk is drawn out to form the thyroglossal duct, and its original site marked on the tongue as the *foramen cecum*. The distal portion of the duct forms the pyramidal lobe of the thyroid, while the remaining duct disappears during Week 5.

By Week 7 the gland has reached its site in the neck. The ultimobranchial body (fourth pharyngeal pouch) fuses with the thyroid and gives rise to parafollicular or 'C' cells in the thyroid. These cells are neural crest derivatives. They store and secrete calcitonin to regulate calcium levels in body fluids. The original solid endodermal mass is infiltrated by vascular mesoderm which breaks the endoderm into plates. By Week 10 the plates have formed cells grouped around a follicle lumen.

Colloid appears in the follicles during Week 11 and thyroxine by Week 18.

- Occasionally, remnants of the midline thyroglossal duct persist and may give rise to aberrant thyroid tissue, sinuses, cysts and fistulae.
- A lingual thyroid may develop if the thyroid has failed to descend.

PARATHYROIDS

The superior parathyroid glands develop from the fourth pharyngeal pouch endoderm. The inferior parathyroid glands develop from the third pharyngeal pouch endoderm. Their primordia appear as buds whose cells form the chief cells, while vascular mesoderm infiltrates the bud to form the capillary network.

The fourth pharyngeal pouch gives rise to the ultimobranchial body, as well as, to the superior parathyroid glands which are found on the posterior surface of the thyroid. The third pharyngeal pouch gives rise to the thymus gland, as well as, the inferior parathyroid glands. As the thymus gland migrates the inferior parathyroids are carried caudally to a final position on the posterior thyroid surface inferior to the superior parathyroids.

During Week 12 parathyroid hormone is produced and is believed to play a role in fetal calcium metabolism.

- Between birth and puberty the parathyroids double in size.

108a	**108b and c**
1. mandibular prominence	**1.** common carotid artery
2. thorax	**2.** cricoid cartilage
3. thymus primordia	**3.** inferior thyroid veins
4. thyroid primordium	**4.** isthmus of thyroid
	5. lobe of thyroid gland
	6. sternocleidomastoid muscle

108a–108f. Thyroid development. View of the ventral (front) surface.

108a. Stages 16–18 (Days 37–44). The early thyroid, view of the right side. 14 mm CR

108b. Stage 19 (Days 47–48). 20 mm CR

108c. Week 9. 50 mm CR ♀

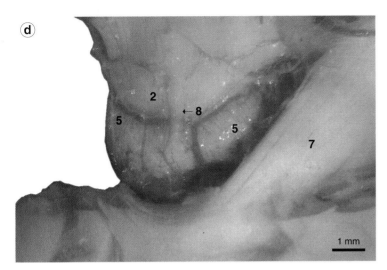

108d. Week 12. Viewed from the left and front. 85 mm CR ♀

108e. Week 13. 97 mm CR ♂

108f. Week 13.
101 mm CR ♀

1. chin
2. cricoid cartilage
3. inferior thyroid veins
4. isthmus of thyroid
5. lobe of thyroid gland
6. omohyoid muscle
7. sternocleidomastoid muscle
8. thyroglossal duct

109. Week 12. Transverse section of thyroid gland. 85 mm CR

1. colloid
2. cuboidal epithelium

109 from QUB

110. Week 13. Dorsum of the tongue to illustrate the *foramen cecum.* 100 mm CR ♀

1. arytenoid swelling
2. epiglottis
3. lip
4. sulcus terminalis
5. vallate papillae

Thymus

The thymus develops when two bilateral masses from the third pharyngeal pouch fuse in the midline. This fused endodermal mass with the adjacent mesoderm and neural crest cells are infiltrated by lymphoid stem cells by Week 10. Epithelial cells derived from the endoderm form the thymic Hassall's corpuscles and cytoreticulum.

After Week 10 young lymphocytes from the thymus circulate in the blood stream and 'seed' the spleen, lymph nodes, and Peyer's patches, where they multiply.

The thymus is prominent and occupies a large part of the superior mediastinum.

- In the neonate the most common form is a bilobar thymus, though it may be trilobar or have no definite lobulation.
- The maximum size occurs at around 12 years in females and 14 years in males.
- After puberty, the thymus becomes infiltrated with fat and in old age is present as a small mass of fibrous tissue.

111a–111h. Ventral view of the developing thymus.

111a. Stages 16–17 (Days 37–41). 12 mm CR

111b. Stages 16–18 (Days 37–44). 14 mm CR

111c. Week 9. 48 mm CR

111d. Week 9. 50 mm CR

111e. Week 10. 57 mm CR ♂

111f. Week 11. 62 mm CR ♂

1.	atrium
2.	diaphragm
3.	liver
4.	lung
5.	pericardium
6.	phrenic nerve
7.	rib
8.	sympathetic chain
9.	thymus
10.	ventricle

(g)

111g. Week 15. 123 mm CR ♀

1. anterior interventricular branch of left coronary artery and great cardiac vein
2. lung
3. pericardium
4. rib
5. thymus
6. ventricle

111h. Week 17. View of the right side of the developing thymus. 152 mm CR ♂

111i. Stage 23 (Days 56–57). Transverse section through the developing manubrium sterni and thymus gland. 28 mm CR

1. clavicle
2. thymus
3. two sternal bars of manubrium sterni

111j. Week 8. Transverse section through the thymus gland. 40 mm CR

111i from LHSM

111j from St T

Thorax

112a–112j. Changes in dissected specimens of the thorax and abdomen.

112a–112c. Lateral view.

112a. Stage 17 (Day 41). 12 mm CR

1. arm	
2. diaphragm	
3. head	
4. heart	
5. intestine	
6. leg	
7. liver	
8. lung	
9. mesonephroi	
10. stomach	
11. thymus	
12. umbilical cord	

General body plan

The early trunk and abdomen (Week 6) are dominated by the appearance of the heart and liver. As the fetus develops, these two organs decrease in size relative to the rest of the body.

- At birth the right side of the liver is larger than the left side due to preferential growth.

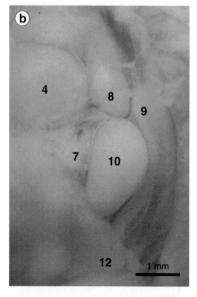

112b. Stages 17–18 (Days 41–44). 14 mm CR

112c. Stage 19 (Days 47–48). 20 mm CR

112d–112j. Ventral view.

112d. Week 8. 34 mm CR

112e. Week 9. 48 mm CR ?

112f. Week 9. 50 mm CR /

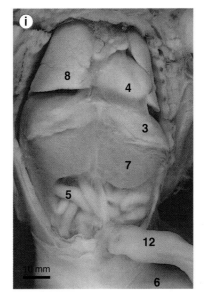

1. arm
2. brain
3. diaphragm
4. heart
5. intestine
6. leg
7. liver
8. lung
9. nose
10. thymus
11. tongue
12. umbilical cord
13. vertebral column

112g. Week 11. 65 mm CR ♂

112h. Week 13. 92 mm CR ♀

112i. Week 13. 101 mm CR ♀

112j. Week 18. 152 mm CR ♂

113. Week 22. A median sagittal section to illustrate the position of vital organs. 159 mm CR

113 from RFHSM

Heart

The heart develops from splanchnopleuric mesoderm, which forms a horseshoe-shaped area in the anterior part of the embryonic disc. Two midline endothelial tubes form (Days 18–19) from this region and fuse to form a single heart tube at Day 22. The two umbilical veins open into the caudal (venous) end of the heart tube, while the two primitive aortae open from the cephalic (arterial) end. The surrounding splanchnopleuric mesoderm condenses to form the myoepicardial mantle. Between the heart tube and mantle tube connective tissue forms cardiac jelly, which develops into subendocardial tissue. The inner tube will form the endocardium, while the outer tube will form the myocardium and epicardium. As the head fold forms, the heart tube comes to lie dorsal to the coelom and ventral to the gut. A dorsal mesentery (mesocardium) suspends the heart. Later, a passage (the transverse sinus) forms through this dorsal mesocardium.

The heart tube divides into bulges: these in cephalic to caudal order are bulbus cordis, primitive ventricle, and atrium. The truncus arteriosus is soon recognizable cranial to the bulbus cordis and is continuous with the aortic sac. The sinus venosus appears inferior to the atrium and has two horns, each formed by the confluence of one common cardinal, one umbilical, and one vitelline vein.

As the heart tube continues to grow, a 'U' shaped bulboventricular loop forms from the primitive ventricle, and the bulbus cordis bulges to the left and cranially. As the loop forms, the atrium is carried cephalic to the bulboventricular loop and comes to lie closely apposed to it. The sinus venosus is carried cranially to lie dorsal to the atrium. The primitive atrium expands to the right and left. The division between the bulbus cordis and ventricle is lost and a single ventricular chamber is formed.

The heart begins to contract by Day 22 and an ebb-and-flow circulation is established. By the end of Week 4 the circulation is unidirectional. The heart is divided internally between Weeks 4 and 5.

1. arm bud
2. atrium
3. auricular appendage
4. back
5. bulbus cordis
6. common carotid artery
7. eye
8. forebrain
9. hand plate (paddle)
10. heart
11. leg bud
12. liver
13. lung
14. mouth
15. pulmonary trunk
16. truncus arteriosus
17. umbilical cord
18. ventricle

114a–114f. External features of the developing heart.

114a. Stage 17 (Day 41). The heart *in situ*, viewed from the left. 12 mm CR

114b. Stages 16–17 (Days 37–41). The ventricles are a single chamber, viewed from the ventral surface. 12 mm CR

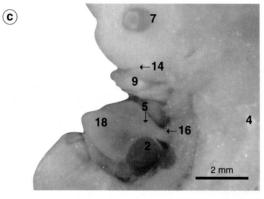

114c. Stage 19 (Days 47–48). Two ventricles are present, viewed from the left. The left arm has been removed. 20 mm CR

114d. The same embryo as in **114c**, view of the right side.

114e. Week 9. The heart and lungs dissected from the specimen, view of the ventral surface. 48 mm CR

114f. Week 10. The dissected heart, viewed from the left. 57 mm CR

115a–115c. A series of developing hearts from the ventral surface.

1. aorta
2. atrium
3. auricle
4. great cardiac vein and anterior interventricular artery
5. pulmonary trunk
6. superior vena cava
7. ventricle

115a. Week 9. 48 mm CR   **115b.** Week 13. 92 mm CR ♀   **115c.** Week 15. 123 mm CR ♀

116a and **116b.** Week 10. The heart *in situ* with pericardium and following its removal. 56 mm CR

1. auricle
2. diaphragm
3. liver
4. lung
5. pericardium
6. thymus
7. ventricle

116a. With pericardium.   **116b.** Pericardium removed.

117a and **117b.** Week 13. The blood supply to the heart's external surface. 92 mm CR ♀

117a. View of the ventral surface.

117b. View of the dorsal surface.

1. auricle
2. coronary sinus
3. great cardiac vein and anterior interventricular artery
4. inferior vena cava
5. middle cardiac vein
6. posterior vein of the left ventricle
7. pulmonary vein
8. ventricle

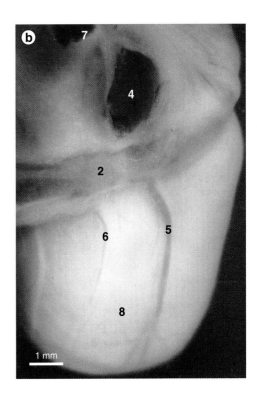

ATRIUM

Partition of atrioventricular canal

Endocardial cushions form in the atrioventricular canal on the dorsal and ventral walls. During Week 5 the cushions grow toward each other, fuse (atrioventricular cushion), and divide the canal into right and left halves.

Partition of primitive atrium

The sinus venosus opens into the future right atrium. Right and left venous valves form on either side of the sinus venous opening, and two valves fuse cephalic to the sinus venosus as the septum spurium. In Week 6 a midline crescent-shaped septum, septum primum, forms on the dorsal atrial wall. This septum grows toward the ventral wall, completely dividing the primitive atrium into two atria and fusing with the atrioventricular cushion. As septum primum approaches the cushion, the opening (foramen primum) becomes progressively smaller. As the septum primum fuses with the left side of the cushion, foramen primum disappears and the foramen secundum forms in the septum primum near its dorsal margin.

At the end of Week 5, the septum secundum appears on the ventrocranial wall and grows in a crescent shape toward the dorsocaudal wall between the septum primum and the septum spurium. This septum is an incomplete partition leaving an opening, the foramen ovale. The septum primum degenerates at its dorsal point of origin and the remainder of the septum forms the valve of the foramen ovale.

Sinus venosus

All venous blood enters the right atrium through the sinus venosus, which has equally-sized right and left horns. During Week 4 the right horn enlarges and the left horn becomes a tributary, which will form the coronary sinus. These changes are the result of two left-to-right shunts of blood (see Blood vessels). As the atrium grows it incorporates the right sinus venosus into its dorsal wall. The right anterior and common cardinal veins form the superior vena cava, the right vitelline vein the terminal part of the inferior vena cava, and the right umbilical vein regresses and disappears. The greater part of the atrium is derived from the sinus venosus and is smooth-walled. The primitive atrium forms the auricle and has musculi pectinati in its walls.

The septum spurium and upper part of the right venous valve together form the crista terminalis. The lower part of the right venous valve forms the valves of the inferior vena cava and coronary sinus.

The single pulmonary vein opens into the left atrium. As the atrium grows it incorporates the pulmonary vein and its four tributaries (two to each lung) into its walls. This part of the atrium is smooth-walled, while the part derived from the primitive atrium has musculi pectinati in its walls.

118a. Stages 12–13 (Days 25–28). Transverse section through the early heart. 5 mm CR

118a from the Boyd Collection

1. atrium
2. dorsal aorta
3. neural tube
4. notochord
5. tracheoesophageal tube
6. ventricle

118b. Stages 15–16 (Days 33–39). Transverse section through the early ventricle. 10 mm CR

1. conus swellings
2. medial nasal prominence
3. ventricle

119a and **119b.** Stage 19 (Days 47–48). The septum primum, viewed through the opened left atrium. 20 mm CR ♀

1. aorta
2. developing septum primum
3. left atrium with fused endocardial cushions
4. left ventricle
5. pulmonary trunk

119c and **119d.** Week 13. The left atrium opened on the dorsal (back) surface to illustrate the septae. The area between the two septae has been artificially enlarged. 92 mm CR ♀

1. coronary sinus
2. foramen ovale (enlarged)
3. left atrium
4. middle cardiac vein
5. right atrium
6. septum primum
7. septum secundum
8. ventricle

VENTRICLE

Partition of primitive ventricle

The primitive ventricle is divided into right and left halves by an interventricular septum arising from the floor near the apex of the primitive ventricle. This crescent-shaped septum grows cranially toward the atrioventricular cushion. An interventricular foramen between the edge of the interventricular septum and fused endocardial cushions disappears during Week 7 when the right bulbar ridge, left bulbar ridge and atrioventricular cushion tissue fuse.

Ventricular walls

A sponge-work of muscle bundles is formed, some of which form trabeculae carneae, and others the papillary muscles and chordae tendineae.

Partition of bulbus cordis and truncus arteriosus

During Week 5 two ridges appear opposite to one another in the bulbus cordis and truncus arteriosus, which spiral inferiorly toward the heart. These ridges fuse (spiral septum) in the midline and divide the bulbus cordis and truncus arteriosus into two vessels, the aorta and the pulmonary trunk. The bulbus cordis is eventually incorporated into the ventricles, the infundibulum into the right ventricle, and the aortic vestibule into the left ventricle.

Cardiac valves

The semilunar valves of the aorta and pulmonary trunk form from the three subendocardial swellings. These swellings hollow out and form cusps. The tricuspid and mitral valves form similarly.

Conducting system

The sinoatrial node forms in the right wall of the sinus venosus and is incorporated into the right atrium. Cells from the left wall of the sinus venosus are incorporated into the interatrial septum and, with cells from the atrioventricular canal region, are known as the atrioventricular node and bundle of His.

120a and 120b. Stage 19 (Days 47–48). The ventricle, viewed from the left. The wall has been dissected. 20 mm CR

1. aorta
2. auricle
3. interventricular foramen
4. left atrium
5. left ventricle
6. pulmonary trunk
7. trabeculae carneae

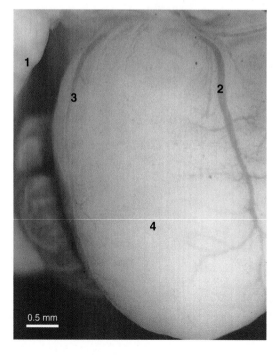

121. Week 9. Blood supply of the dorsal surface of the heart. 48 mm CR ♀

1. lung
2. middle cardiac vein and posterior interventricular branch of right coronary artery
3. posterior vein of left ventricle
4. ventricle

FETAL CIRCULATION

Oxygenated blood from the placenta returns to the fetus via the umbilical vein, which enters the fetus to become the left umbilical vein.

Some of the oxygenated blood passes through the hepatic sinusoids and some bypasses the liver via the ductus venosus and enters the inferior vena cava, where it mixes with venous blood from the fetal lower limbs, pelvis, and abdomen. This blood enters the right atrium and is directed toward the foramen ovale by the valve of the inferior vena cava. The lower border of the septum secundum (crista dividens) deflects the flow into two unequal streams. The larger flow passes through the foramen ovale; the lesser flow mixes with the venous return through the superior vena cava and passes through to the right ventricle, where it is passed to the pulmonary artery, ductus arteriosus, descending aorta, and returns to the placenta via the umbilical arteries. Some is also distributed to the viscera. Little passes to the lungs because of the high pulmonary vascular resistance.

The main stream passing through the foramen ovale to the left atrium mixes with any blood returning from the lungs, enters the left ventricle and then the ascending aorta which distributes to the head, neck, and upper limbs.

CHANGES AT BIRTH

At birth the foramen ovale, ductus arteriosus, ductus venosus, umbilical arteries, and umbilical vein become no longer functional.

With the interruption to placental circulation, there is a drop in blood pressure in the inferior vena cava and right atrium. As the lungs are aerated and the pulmonary blood flow greatly increased, the pressure in the left atrium is greater than that in the right atrium. This increased pressure presses the septum primum against the septum secundum and closes the foramen ovale.

The ductus arteriosis constricts at birth as do the umbilical arteries. The cord is usually not tied for a minute or two to allow blood in the placenta to return to the neonate via the umbilical vein.

Later the ductus arteriosus, ductus venosus, and the umbilical vessels are occluded by proliferation of endothelial and fibrous tissue.

The umbilical vein is discernible as the ligamentum teres, which usually retains a reduced but patent lumen, even in the adult.

The umbilical arteries remain distally as the medial umbilical ligaments; proximally, they remain patent and give off the superior vesical arteries.

The ligamentum venosum is the remnant of the ductus venosus.

In the heart, the septum primum forms the floor of the fossa ovalis, while the lower margin of the septum secundum forms the annulus ovalis.

The ductus arteriosus forms the ligamentum arteriosum. The ductus is obliterated by tissue by the end of the third month after birth.

122a and **122b.** The ductus arteriosus viewed from the left. Left lung removed.

122a. Week 15. 123 mm CR ♀

122b. Week 18. 152 mm CR ♂

1. arch of aorta
2. auricular appendage of the heart
3. common carotid artery
4. descending aorta
5. ductus arteriosus
6. intercostal vessels
7. left subclavian artery
8. right lung
9. sympathetic trunk
10. thymus gland
11. trachea
12. ventricle of the heart

Circulatory system

BLOOD AND BLOOD VESSELS

The first blood and blood vessels develop from angioblasts (mesoderm) on the yolk sac, connecting stalk, and in the chorion during Stages 6–8 (Days 13–15). In Week 3 small groups of angioblasts form blood islands in the yolk sac and body stalk. In each island spaces appear and the central cells form nucleated primitive red blood cells and the peripheral ones the vascular endothelium of the blood vessels. Later, several islands join together to form vessels. Mesoderm surrounding the vessels will form the connective tissue and muscular elements of the vessels.

As blood islands are established in the liver (Week 5), spleen (Week 10), and bone marrow (Weeks 9–12) the extra-embryonic hemopoietic supply disappears (Week 6). After birth, only the bone marrow normally continues as an hemopoietic organ.

Fetal blood does not coagulate until Weeks 10–12. Before the end of Week 3 two endothelial heart tubes form similarly, fuse to form a single heart tube, and by Day 20 have linked up with the blood vessels of the embryo, allantois, and yolk sac. By the end of Week 3 the cardiovascular system is established and the heart is contracting from the sinus venosus. By the end of Week 4 the contractions have established a unidirectional flow.

Blood returns to the heart from the embryo via the anterior and posterior common cardinal veins, from the placenta via the umbilical veins, and from the yolk sac via the vitelline veins. All three vessels on each side join at the septum transversum and enter the heart.

Blood leaves the heart to the body via the aortic arches to the paired dorsal aortae which form a single vessel posteriorly, to the placenta via the umbilical arteries, and to the yolk sac via the vitelline arteries.

- While the neonatal kidney adjusts functionally during the first week after birth the blood urea is slightly high.
- Fetal hemoglobin predominates at birth.

ARTERIES

Each branchial arch is supplied by an artery arising from the aortic sac and passing to its respective right or left aorta. The arteries are not all present at the same time; the first two degenerate before the last appears, and the fifth is rudimentary. By Stages 13–14 (Days 28–30) the dorsal aortae are extended cranially to form the internal carotids, and from the sixth arch artery a branch called the pulmonary artery supplies each lung bud. The first and second arch arteries develop into the maxillary and stapedial arteries respectively.

Carotid arteries

The common carotids form from the third aortic arches. Where the third and fourth arch arteries are connected to one another by sections of aortae, these segments disappear to leave the original third arch arteries to form the proximal internal carotids and the aortae to form the distal portions. The internal carotids give off anterior and middle cerebral branches and an ophthalmic branch to the optic vesicle. The external carotids may receive a contribution from the roots of the first arch arteries.

Umbilical arteries

At birth, the umbilical arteries become non-functional, but remain patent at the proximal end where each has a superior vesicular branch to supply the bladder.

Vitelline arteries

The vitelline arteries disappear and a new vessel forms a single superior mesenteric artery supplying the midgut. Later, the celiac artery will form to supply the foregut and the inferior mesenteric to supply the hindgut.

Intersegmental arteries

There are approximately 30 pairs of intersegmental arteries arising from the dorsal aortae. They pass successively between the somites. In the neck they join together to form the vertebral artery. In the thorax and abdomen they are retained as the intercostal arteries and lumbar arteries respectively. The right seventh intersegmental artery contributes to the right subclavian, while the left seventh intersegmental artery forms the left subclavian of the adult. The fifth lumbar arteries with the umbilical arteries form the common iliac arteries.

Pulmonary trunk

As the spiral ridges divide the truncus arteriosus (see Heart) two vessels are formed; the pulmonary trunk and the ascending aorta. As this division extends into the aortic sac, the sixth arch artery connects to the pulmonary trunk and the remaining vessels to the aorta.

Aorta

The left half of the truncus arteriosus forms the ascending aorta; the fourth arch artery forms the arch of the aorta and the left dorsal aorta forms the descending aorta. The distal part of the sixth arch artery forms the ductus arteriosus (see Changes at birth).

123. Stages 15–16 (Days 33–37). Transverse section of the aorta with blood cells. 9 mm CR

123 from QUB

1. aorta
2. mesoderm
3. nucleated red blood cells
4. vascular endothelium

1 mm

124. Stages 16–17 (Days 37–41). Yolk sac of the early embryo. 12 mm CR

1. amnion
2. forebrain
3. umbilical cord
4. yolk sac

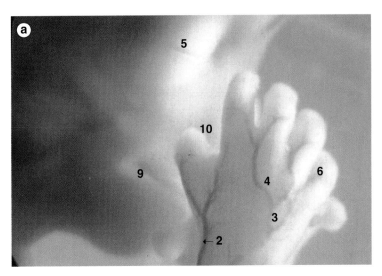

125a. Week 9. The dorsal venous network. 53 mm CR

125a–125c. Blood vessels developing in the limbs. Note the thin layer of skin over the vessels.

1 mm

125b. Week 9. Great saphenous vein of the leg. 48 mm CR

125c. Week 12. The dorsal venous network of the foot. 85 mm CR

1. ankle
2. cephalic vein
3. dorsal venous network
4. dorsum of hand
5. eye
6. finger (minimus)
7. great saphenous vein
8. knee
9. mouth
10. nose
11. toes

126a. Arteriogram of a 122 mm CR fetus, anteroposterior view. .

1. abdominal aorta
2. anterior tibial
3. axillary
4. basilar
5. brachial
6. common carotid
7. deep palmar arch
8. dorsalis pedis
9. external carotid
10. external iliac
11. femoral
12. heart
13. internal carotid
14. lung
15. middle cerebral
16. popliteal
17. posterior tibial
18. radial
19. right pulmonary
20. subclavian
21. superior mesenteric
22. ulnar
23. umbilical
24. vertebral

5 mm

126a from Mr J. Bashford and Mr R.H. Watts, J.D. Boyd and W.J. Hamilton Collections

126b. Arteriogram of a 170 mm CR fetus, lateral view.

1. abdominal aorta
2. anterior tibial
3. common carotid
4. dorsalis pedis
5. external carotid
6. external iliac
7. femoral
8. internal carotid
9. popliteal
10. posterior tibial
11. radial
12. superior mesenteric
13. ulnar
14. umbilical
15. vertebral

126b from Mr J. Bashford, J.D. Boyd

127. Cast of the arterial supply of the fetus.

1. anterior tibial
2. axillary
3. clavicle bone
4. common carotid
5. external iliac
6. femoral
7. femur (broken) bone
8. humerus (broken) bone
9. internal thoracic
10. lung
11. mandible bone
12. orbit bones
13. popliteal
14. posterior tibial
15. radial
16. tibia bone

10 mm

127 from RFHSM

128. Resin cast of the arterial supply of the kidneys and lower limbs, viewed from behind.

1. anterior tibial artery
2. aorta
3. femoral artery
4. femur
5. kidney
6. liver
7. popliteal artery
8. suprarenal (adrenal) gland
9. tibia
10. umbilical arteries

10 mm

128 from RFHSM

VEINS

Anterior cardinal veins

Blood drains from three plexi in the head into the anterior (pre-)cardinal veins. The superficial vessels of the plexi form dural venous sinuses and the deep vessels form the cerebral veins.

Common cardinal veins

The anterior and posterior cardinal veins join to form the common cardinal veins lying in the septum transversum and opening into the sinus venosus. The right common cardinal vein forms the superior vena cava, while the left becomes a tributary of the coronary sinus.

Posterior cardinal veins

The posterior cardinal veins drain the body walls, spinal cord, and mesonephroi. They are obliterated largely by the mesonephroi pressing against them, and are replaced by a new pair of subcardinal veins. These lie medial to the mesonephroi and connect with the subcardinal anastomosis.

A new channel (subcardinal vitelline anastomosis) forms to connect the stump of the right vitelline vein to the subcardinal vein. This channel, together with the right subcardinal, sacrocardinal segment, and right vitelline, forms the inferior vena cava.

Finally, the supracardinals appear, become broken up in the region of the kidneys, unite by an anastomosis, and form the azygos and hemiazygos vessels. The root of the azygos vein forms from the right posterior cardinal vein.

Umbilical and vitelline veins

On each side the umbilical and vitelline veins pass through the septum transversum and enter the sinus venosus. Where the vessels cross the septum transversum they become invested by the liver cords and form hepatic sinuses. Caudal to this region the right umbilical vein atrophies in Week 6. Cranial to the liver sinusoids the right and left umbilical veins and the left vitelline vein atrophy. Blood from the placenta flows via the left umbilical vein into the septum transversum where a shunt, the ductus venosus, connects the flow to the right vitelline vein, which has enlarged to form the hepatocardiac channel.

At birth the placental flow ceases and the left umbilical vein becomes the ligamentum teres, while the ductus venosus becomes the ligamentum venosum. The hepatic sinusoids drain into the right hepatocardiac channel which forms the terminal part of the inferior vena cava.

Portal vein

Caudal to the liver, three sets of vessels develop to connect the two vitelline veins. The cranial and caudal anastomosing vessels pass ventrally and the middle passes dorsally to the duodenum. The portal vein forms when the left vitelline vein disappears between the cranial and middle anastomoses and the right vitelline vein disappears between the middle and caudal anastomoses. The intrahepatic portion of the portal vein forms from hepatic sinusoids derived from the vitelline vein.

The vitello-intestinal duct and caudal parts of the vitelline vein degenerate concomitantly.

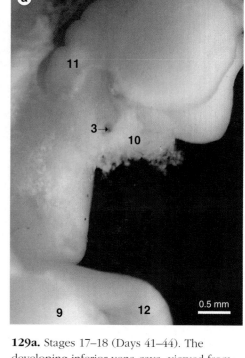

129a. Stages 17–18 (Days 41–44). The developing inferior vena cava, viewed from the right. 14 mm CR

129b. A resin cast of the blood supply to the developing liver.

129c. Week 10. The blood vessels dissected out of the developing liver, viewed from the dorsal (back) surface. 60 mm CR

1. caudate lobe
2. common iliac veins
3. developing inferior vena cava
4. ductus venosus
5. inferior vena cava
6. kidney
7. left hepatic vein
8. left lobe of liver
9. leg bud (right)
10. liver cords (liver dissected off)
11. lung bud
12. midgut herniation
13. portal sinus
14. portal vein
15. quadrate lobe
16. right hepatic vein
17. right lobe of liver
18. umbilical vein

129b from RCS

130a–130g. Development of the lungs.

130a. Stages 17–18 (Days 41–44). Right lung, viewed *in situ*.
14 mm CR

Lungs

A respiratory (laryngotracheal) diverticulum forms in the floor of the pharynx at Day 26. Two endodermal bronchial buds grow from the caudal end of this bulb-shaped diverticulum, or lung bud (Day 28), and are surrounded by splanchnic mesoderm. These two components will form the lung. The cephalic end of the diverticulum will form the trachea. During Week 5 the smaller left bronchial bud divides into two secondary bronchi and the right into three secondary bronchi, which correspond with the main bronchi and lobes of the adult lung. Early in development the right main bronchus is more vertical than the left. Each bronchus then subdivides several times (Weeks 7–24) to form a bronchial tree.

Breathing movements occur before birth, which draw amniotic fluid into the lungs. Fluid from the lungs and tracheal glands is also present in the airways. Fetal breathing movements are detectable using ultrasonography. These movements are essential for normal lung development and allow the fetus to practice and exercise the respiratory muscles.

At birth, the first breath must overcome both the elastic resistance of the lungs themselves and the surface tension of the fluid in the lungs. The alveoli near the bronchi dilate, while those at the periphery expand by Days 3–4 of postnatal development. The neonate has one-eighth to one-sixth of the adult number of alveoli. Alveoli continue to form until approximately 8 years of age.

130b. The lung buds shown in **130a** dissected from the embryo. The lungs already show the adult pattern of lobes.

1. left main bronchus
2. liver cords
3. pericardium
4. pleural membrane
5. right lung
6. right main bronchus
7. trachea
8. ventricles of the heart
9. inferior lobe left lung
10. superior lobe left lung
11. inferior lobe right lung
12. middle lobe right lung
13. superior lobe right lung

- A natural 'detergent' or surfactant is secreted in the lungs from Week 20 and can reduce the surface tension of the fluids which line the airways. Hyaline membrane disease, which is associated with a deficiency or absence of surfactant, is a common cause of death in infants born before Week 32. Thyroxine and glucocorticoid treatments stimulate surfactant production.
- The fluid-filled lungs of a stillborn infant will sink at autopsy when placed in water. Lungs of an infant which has drawn breath will float. This fact may be of medico-legal importance.
- After birth a foreign body is more likely to enter the right main bronchus than the left, because of the more vertical direction of the right bronchus.

130c. Stages 18–19 (Days 44–48). Coronal section of the lungs and heart. 17 mm CR

130c from QUB

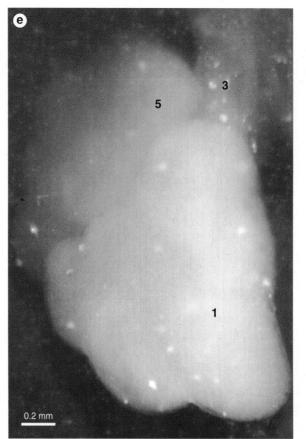

1. inferior lobe left lung
2. inferior lobe right lung
3. left main bronchus
4. middle lobe right lung
5. superior lobe left lung
6. superior lobe right lung
7. trachea

0.5 mm

0.2 mm

130d. Stage 19 (Days 47–48). Dissection of early lung, viewed from the back (dorsal) surface. 20 mm CR

130e. The left lung in **130d** at a higher magnification, viewed from the back.

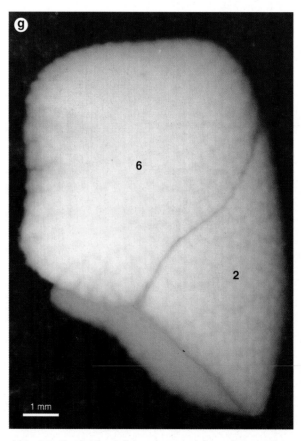

1. auricle of the heart
2. inferior lobe left lung
3. inferior lobe right lung
4. lobules
5. middle lobe right lung
6. superior lobe left lung
7. superior lobe right lung

0.5 mm

1 mm

130f. Week 9. The right lung, viewed from the diaphragmatic surface. Note the lobules. 48 mm CR ♀

130g. Week 10. The left lung, viewed from the costal surface. 56 mm CR

131a and **131b.** Development of the lungs as viewed from the back (dorsal) surface.

1. inferior lobe left lung
2. inferior lobe right lung
3. left main bronchus
4. middle lobe right lung
5. superior lobe left lung
6. superior lobe right lung
7. trachea

131a. Week 9. 48 mm CR ♂

131b. Week 10. 60 mm CR ♀

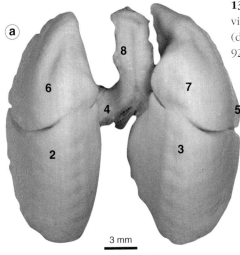

132a. Week 13. Lungs, viewed from the back (dorsal) surface. 92 mm CR ♀

1. diaphragmatic surface
2. inferior lobe left lung
3. inferior lobe right lung
4. left main bronchus
5. middle lobe right lung
6. superior lobe left lung
7. superior lobe right lung
8. trachea

132b. The same lungs as in **132a**, viewed from the ventral and diaphragmatic surface.

133a–133c. The trachea.

133a. Stage 22 (Day 54). Coronal section of the bifurcation of the trachea. 25 mm CR

1. cartilage
2. cilia
3. left main bronchus
4. lung
5. mesenchyme cells
6. microvilli
7. right main bronchus
8. trachea

133b. Week 12. Longitudinal section of a tracheal cartilage ring, viewed by scanning electron microscopy. 80 mm CR

133c. Week 12. Tracheal epithelium, viewed by scanning electron microscopy. 80 mm CR

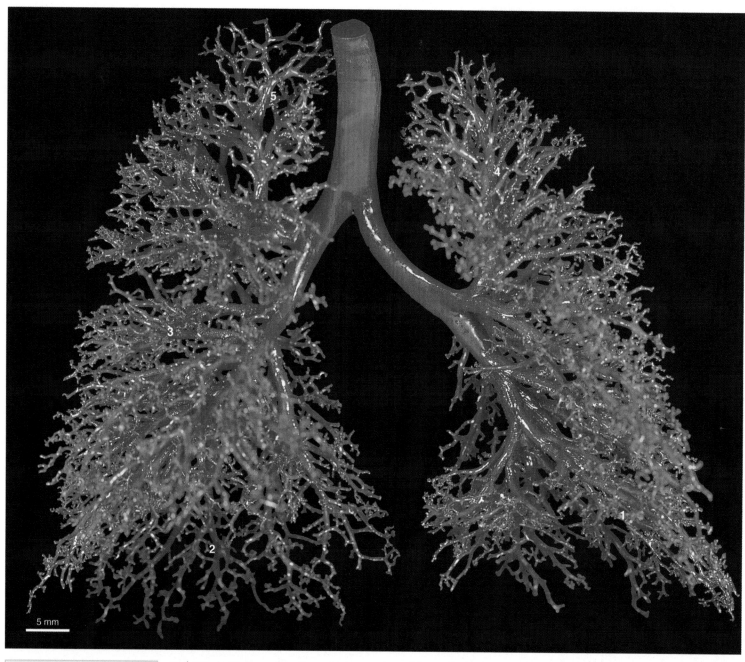

1. inferior lobe left lung
2. inferior lobe right lung
3. middle lobe right lung
4. superior lobe left lung
5. superior lobe right lung

134. Week 30. Cast of the bronchial tree, viewed from the front (ventral) surface.

134 from RCS

FOUR STAGES OF DEVELOPMENT

There are four overlapping stages of lung development, spanning the embryonic to the childhood periods.

In the Pseudoglandular Period (Weeks 5–17) the lung resembles a gland. Structures necessary for gaseous exchange have not yet formed, and hence survival is not possible.

In the Canalicular Period (Weeks 16–25) the lung tissue becomes highly vascularized; respiratory bronchioles, alveolar ducts, and some primitive alveoli (terminal sacs) have formed. Survival is possible with intensive care.

In the Terminal Sac Period (Week 24 to Birth) the four requirements for survival are increasingly present: numerous thin terminal sacs form which can provide adequate gaseous exchange; type II cells provide sufficient surfactant; sufficient pulmonary vascularity and pulmonary lymphatics develop.

In the Alveolar Period (late fetal to 8 years) the number of bronchioles and primitive alveoli increases. Approximately 95% of alveoli develop after birth and all mature alveoli form after birth.

135a–135d. Early development of the lung.

135a. Stages 15–16 (Days 33–37). Lung buds. 10 mm CR

135b. Stages 15–16 (Days 33–37). Transverse section of the lung bud. 10 mm CR

135b from CCHMS

135c. Stage 23 (Days 56–57). 28 mm CR

135c from LHSM

135d. Week 8. Coronal section of lung. 40 mm CR

135d from St T

1. aorta	**7.** lung bud
2. arm bud	**8.** pleural cavity
3. dorsal aortae	**9.** posterior cardinal vein
4. esophagus	**10.** sinus venosus
5. left atrium	**11.** sympathetic trunk
6. lung	**12.** vertebral body

136. Week 13. The lung resembles a gland. 101 mm CR ♀

1. blood vessels
2. bronchi
3. bronchioles
4. early airways

137. Week 20. The lung more closely resembles the neonate lung.

138. Stage 22 (Day 54). Coronal section of trachea and lungs. 25 mm CR.

1. lung
2. primary bronchus
3. trachea

Diaphragm

The diaphragm has several origins; the central tendon from the septum transversum and smaller contributions from the thoracic body wall (costal) and the dorsal mesentery of the esophagus (median portion of the diaphragm) and a dorsolateral part from the pleuroperitoneal membranes.

The muscles of the diaphragm form (Week 5) primarily from the fourth cervical myotome which invades the septum transversum. The phrenic nerve (C3,4,5) is carried with the septum transversum as it migrates caudally. The crura form from myoblasts growing into the dorsal mesentery of the esophagus.

The liver and the enlarging pleural cavities cause the diaphragm to be dome-shaped.

1. atrium
2. cactus needle
3. heart
4. intestine
5. leg bud
6. liver
7. liver removed
8. mesonephroi
9. pleuroperitoneal membrane
10. right lung bud
11. septum transversum
12. stomach

139a–139d. Contributions to the early diaphragm.

139a. Stages 17–18 (Days 41–44). 14 mm CR

139b. Stages 17–18 (Days 41–44). 14 mm CR

139c. Stage 19 (Days 47–48). The liver, viewed from the left side. 20 mm CR

139d. Same embryo as in **139c.** The liver has been removed. No muscle is present yet.

139e–139g. Diaphragm, viewed from below.

139e. Week 8. 34 mm CR

139f. Week 8. 40 mm CR

1. bladder	
2. diaphragm	
3. esophagus	
4. gonad	
5. heart	
6. intestine	
7. lung	
8. stomach	

139g. Week 9. 50 mm CR

139h and **139i.** Diaphragm, viewed from above.

139h. Week 13. 92 mm CR ♂

139i. Week 13. 101 mm CR ♂

139j. Week 18. Phrenic nerve and the diaphragm, viewed from the left. Left lung removed. 152 mm CR

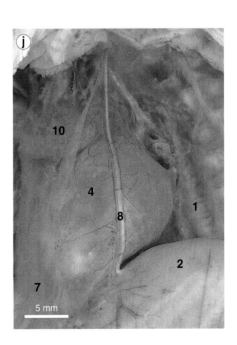

1. aorta	**7.** pericardium
2. diaphragm	**8.** phrenic nerve
3. esophagus	**9.** spinal cord
4. heart	**10.** thymus
5. inferior vena cava	**11.** vertebral body
6. leg	

Abdomen

Body wall

Initially, the anterior abdominal wall is a thin layer of epithelium and mesoderm over the developing organs.

Muscles are formed from myotomes, which are originally on the back (dorsal) and migrate as two sheets around the body on to the ventral surface.

In Week 12 the two sheets fuse in the midline, initially in the upper thoracic and suprapubic regions and then in the abdominal region. Their join is marked as the linea alba.

1. arm
2. genital tubercle
3. head
4. leg bud (leg)
5. linea alba
6. ribs
7. tail
8. umbilical cord

140a–140d. Body wall, view of the abdomen from the cephalic aspect.

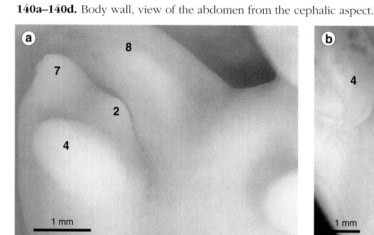

140a. Stages 16–17 (Days 37–41). 12 mm CR

140b. Stage 22 (Day 54). 27 mm CR

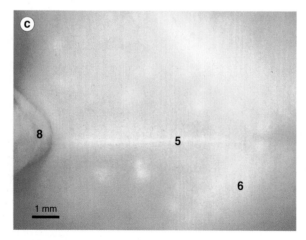

140c. Week 9. 46 mm CR

140d. Week 10. 57 mm CR

Esophagus

The esophagus and trachea are separated as the laryngotracheal (respiratory) diverticulum is pinched off caudally.

The esophagus is a short endodermal tube (Week 4) (see Yolk sac) surrounded by mesoderm which will condense to form the muscle and submucosal layers. By Week 7 the esophagus has elongated owing to the descent of the heart and lungs. The endoderm of the tube proliferates and almost obliterates the lumen; later (Week 8) it recanalizes. The lining of the esophagus is ciliated at Week 11 and loses most of its cilia by Week 28.

- The mainly striated muscle of the upper esophagus forms from the caudal branchial arches and is supplied by the vagus nerve. The mainly non-striated muscles of the lower esophagus develop from the splanchnic mesoderm.
- The esophagus of the neonate may have patches of ciliated columnar cells which disappear rapidly after birth.
- The upper end of the esophagus of the neonate is at the level of C4–C6 and the lower end is at the level of T9. These levels are approximately two vertebrae higher than in the adult.

141a–141d. Development of the esophagus, viewed from the left.

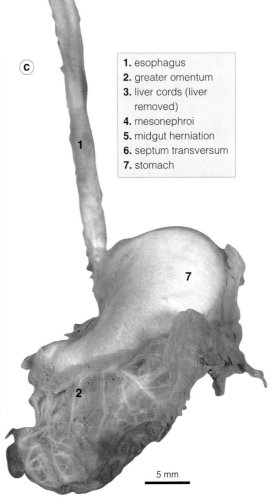

1. esophagus
2. greater omentum
3. liver cords (liver removed)
4. mesonephroi
5. midgut herniation
6. septum transversum
7. stomach

0.5 mm

1 mm

141a. Stages 17–18 (Days 41–44). 14 mm CR

141b. Week 8. Viewed from the front. 40 mm CR

141c. Week 17. 150 mm CR ♀

5 mm

141d. Week 8. A transverse section of the esophagus and trachea. 40 mm CR

141d *from St T*

1. esophagus
2. trachea

142. Week 12. The epithelium lining the esophagus, viewed by scanning electron microscopy. 80 mm CR

1. cilia

Stomach

At Week 4 the foregut caudal to the esophagus forms a spindle-shaped dilatation which descends into the abdomen by Weeks 6–7. During this descent the stomach broadens and the greater curvature forms on the more rapidly growing dorsal border. The stomach rotates through 90° (Week 6) along its longitudinal axis, so that the original left side of the stomach becomes the ventral surface and the right side the dorsal surface.

The stomach is suspended dorsally by a mesentery, the dorsal mesogastrium. Ventrally, the septum transversum thins to form the ventral mesogastrium.

After rotation of the stomach the dorsal mesogastrium elongates and hangs from the greater curvature as the greater omentum. The lesser sac is the space between the large double-layered greater omentum, and the entrance to the lesser sac is the epiploic foramen. The spleen develops in the double-layered sheet of the dorsal mesogastrium.

At Week 7 mucosal pits are present and by Week 8 gastric glands begin to bud off from the pits. Rennin is present in Week 18.

- Using ultrasonography, a stomach bubble is present in the majority of fetuses.
- The stomach of the neonate has a capacity of 30–35 ml, which increases to 100 ml by the end of the first month.
- The musculature of the fetal stomach contracts during development (Week 11), but does not have true peristaltic activity.

Spleen

The spleen develops from mesoderm in the dorsal mesentery of the stomach. A number of mesodermal masses fuse by Weeks 6–7 to form the spleen, and in Weeks 11–12 lymphoblasts produce lymphocytes. The lobulated spleen is an important site for hemopoiesis. By Weeks 13–20 megakaryocytes, myeloblasts, and erythroblasts are present in the spleen and hemopoiesis reaches a peak.

By Week 28 the major site of erythropoeisis is in the bone marrow and it ceases in the spleen by birth.

- In the neonate the long axis of the spleen is usually vertical or oblique.
- Accessory spleens are a common anomaly and usually occur in the greater omentum.
- A functioning thymus in the fetus and the development of the white pulp of the spleen are directly related.
- The spleen produces lymphocytes throughout life.
- The lobules normally disappear before birth leaving a notched superior border to the spleen.

143a–143c. Stages 17–18 (Days 41–44). Early development of the stomach. 14 mm CR

143a. View from the left.

1. cactus needle
2. dorsal mesentery
3. esophagus
4. leg bud
5. liver cords (liver removed)
6. mesonephroi
7. midgut herniation
8. septum transversum
9. stomach

143b. View from the ventral surface.

143c. View from the left.

143d–143i. Development of the stomach and spleen, viewed from the front.

1. cardia
2. esophagus
3. fundus
4. greater curvature
5. greater omentum
6. intestine
7. lesser curvature
8. pyloric antrum
9. spleen
10. stomach

143d. Week 8. 40 mm CR   **143f.** Week 11. 65 mm CR   **143h.** Week 15. 123 mm CR

143e. Week 8. 48 mm CR   **143g.** Week 13. 92 mm CR   **143i.** Week 18. 152 mm CR

144a–144d. Development of the stomach *in situ*, viewed from the ventral surface.

1. bladder
2. diaphragm
3. gonad
4. intestine
5. kidney
6. liver
7. pin head (dressmaking)
8. spleen
9. stomach
10. suprarenal (adrenal) gland

144a. Stage 19 (Days 47–48). 20 mm CR   **144b.** Week 10. 57 mm CR

144c. Week 11. 65 mm CR   **144d.** Week 15. 123 mm CR

145. Week 13. The greater omentum, viewed from the front. 92 mm CR ♀

1. epiploic foramen (entrance to lesser sac)
2. greater omentum
3. intestine
4. stomach

146. Stage 23 (Days 56–57). Transverse section of the developing stomach. 29 mm CR

1. liver
2. spleen
3. stomach

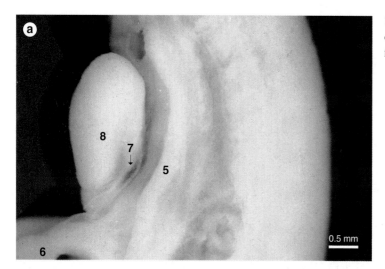

147a. Stages 17–18 (Days 41–44). 14 mm CR

147a–147c. Splenic development, viewed from the left side.

1. body wall
2. greater omentum
3. intestine
4. kidney
5. mesonephroi
6. midgut herniation
7. spleen
8. stomach
9. suprarenal (adrenal) gland

147b. Stage 19 (Days 47–48). The spleen has been reflected medially. 20 mm CR

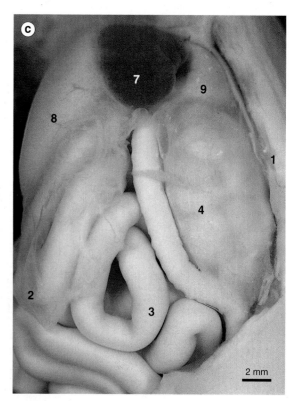

147c. Week 13. 92 mm CR ♀

148. Stages 17–18 (Days 41–44). Early pancreas viewed from the left side. The left leg bud and liver have been removed. 14 mm CR

1. abdomen
2. body wall
3. genital tubercle
4. gonadal ridge
5. mesonephric kidney
6. midgut herniation
7. pancreas primordium (dorsal)
8. stomach

0.5 mm

Pancreas

The pancreas forms during Weeks 5–8 from two endodermal buds of the foregut caudal to the stomach; a large dorsal bud appears first, followed by a smaller, caudal ventral bud. The ventral bud arises on the ventral duodenum near the site of the common bile duct. When the gut rotates (Week 5) the ventral bud is carried medially (clockwise) to fuse with the dorsal bud in the dorsal mesogastrium. Their ducts also anastomose.

The dorsal bud forms part of the head, neck, body, and tail of the pancreas, and the ventral bud part of the head and uncinate process. The duct of the ventral bud and a distal part of the dorsal bud duct form the main pancreatic duct. The proximal part of the dorsal duct may persist as a smaller accessory duct.

The parenchyma, acini, and the islets of Langerhans are endodermal in origin, while the septae and the connective tissue covering are mesodermal. Their development (Week 12) is similar to salivary gland formation.

- Insulin is formed from Week 10.
- There are relatively more islets of Langerhans in the neonate than in the adult.

149a and **149b.** Stage 19 (Days 47–48). The dorsal and ventral pancreatic buds are in contact, viewed from the right side. **149b** is a higher magnification of the embryo in **149a**. 20 mm CR

1. abdomen
2. body wall
3. cactus needle
4. dorsal pancreas
5. gonadal ridge
6. mesonephric kidney
7. midgut
8. stomach
9. ventral pancreas

1 mm

0.5 mm

150a and **150b.** Week 9. The pancreas. **150b** is a higher magnification of the pancreas in **150a**. 45 mm CR

1. caudal
2. cephalic
3. dorsal pancreas
4. intestine
5. kidney
6. liver
7. suprarenal (adrenal) gland
8. ventral pancreas

1 mm

0.5 mm

151. Week 9. The fused pancreatic buds have formed the single pancreas. 48 mm CR ♂

1. intestine
2. pancreas
3. spleen

1 mm

152a and **152b.** Transverse sections of the pancreas.

152a. Stage 22 (Day 54). 25 mm CR

152b. Week 8. 40 mm CR

152 from St T

1. dorsal pancreas	3. liver	5. ventral pancreas
2. intestine	4. pancreas (fused)	

Liver

In Week 4 the liver forms as an endodermal outgrowth (hepatic diverticulum) from the foregut. It penetrates the splanchnic mesoderm of the septum transversum. The hepatic diverticulum then divides (Week 5) into right and left branches, and columns of endodermal cells (liver cords or parenchyma) grow out into the surrounding mesoderm. Sinusoids are formed as the invading liver cells anastomose around endothelium-lined spaces present in the septum transversum. The mesoderm forms the connective and hemopoietic tissue, the Kupffer cells, and the fibrous capsule of the liver. The bile duct system forms when the terminal branches of the right and left hepatic buds canalize.

Initially, the right and left lobes are of equal size, but the right lobe becomes much larger after Week 6 due to relative growth changes. The caudate and quadrate lobes form from the right lobe (Week 6). The liver occupies most of the abdominal cavity at Weeks 6–10.

As the liver enlarges, the yolk sac regresses and hemopoiesis occurs in the liver at Week 6, reaches a peak at Weeks 12–24, but ceases at birth.

Lymphocyte formation occurs in the liver at Week 10, but ceases by birth. Coagulation factors are produced in the liver after Weeks 10–12.

Bile is produced in Week 12.

- Large reserves of carbohydrates are laid down in the liver and skeletal muscle before birth to provide a source of energy for the infant until suckling is well established (around the third day after birth).

Gallbladder

In Week 4 the gallbladder is a solid endodermal outgrowth in continuity with the liver diverticulum. The outgrowth enlarges rapidly and during Weeks 7–8 it canalizes, and forms a sac. The stalk becomes the cystic duct connected to the duodenum via the common bile duct.

Initially, the gallbladder is in the midline, but it becomes more peripheral.

Bile pigment is secreted from Week 13 and colours the colonic contents (meconium) green.

- The neonatal gallbladder is more embedded in the liver substance than it is in the adult, and the fundus often does not extend beyond the margin of the liver.

153. Stage 17 (Day 41). Early liver development, viewed from the left side. 12 mm CR

1. arm bud and hand plate (paddle)
2. branchial arch
3. eye
4. forebrain
5. heart
6. hindbrain
7. leg bud
8. liver
9. umbilical cord

1 mm

0.5 mm

154. Stages 17–18 (Days 41–44). The liver, viewed from the right and front. The skin has been removed. 14 mm CR

1. abdominal cavity
2. arm bud (right)
3. back
4. heart bulge
5. liver

155a–155d. The early liver.

1. arm bud and hand plate with finger rays
2. back
3. eye
4. heart
5. hepato-cardiac veins (vitelline veins)
6. leg bud and foot paddle
7. liver bulge
8. mandibular prominence
9. maxillary prominence
10. midgut herniation
11. septum transversum
12. umbilical cord

155a. Stage 19 (Days 47–48). The liver, viewed from the right and front. 20 mm CR

155b. Higher magnification of the liver in **155a**. The anterior abdominal wall has been dissected off, view from the front.

155c. Stages 15–16 (Days 33–37). A transverse section of the liver. 9 mm CR

155c from QUB

155d. The liver in **155a** dissected from the right side. Note the hepato-cardiac veins.

156a. Stages 17–18 (Days 41–44). The liver, viewed from the left side. Note the liver trabeculae. 14 mm CR

156b. Week 8. The liver, viewed by transmitted light in a fetus cleared in cedarwood oil. 40 mm CR

1. arm bud (left)
2. back
3. body wall
4. leg bud
5. liver cords
6. stomach
7. umbilical cord

1. arm
2. eye
3. leg
4. liver
5. umbilical cord

157a–157c. Transverse paraffin wax sections of the developing liver.

157a–157c from LHSM

157a. Stages 14–15 (Days 32–33). 7 mm CR

157b. Stage 23 (Days 56–57). 28 mm CR

157c. Higher magnification of the liver posterior to the section in **157b.**

1. body wall	**4.** liver	**7.** tributary of hepatic vein	**10.** umbilical vein
2. diaphragm	**5.** lungs	**8.** spinal cord	**11.** vertebral body
3. esophagus	**6.** rib	**9.** stomach	

158a–158d. Full term fetus. Two transverse sections through the upper abdomen.

158a and **158b.** Specimens viewed from above (the superior surface).

1. anterior abdominal wall
2. kidney
3. large intestine
4. liver
5. small intestine
6. spleen
7. stomach
8. vertebral body

158c and **158d.** The same specimens, viewed from below (the inferior surface).

158a–158d from RFHSM

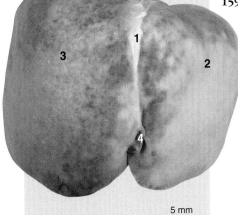

159a–159c. Liver development. The dissected livers are viewed from the ventral surface.

159a. Week 9. 48 mm CR

159b. Week 11. 65 mm CR ♂

159c. Week 13. 92 mm CR ♀

1. falciform ligament
2. left lobe
3. right lobe
4. umbilical vein

160a and **160b.** The course of the umbilical vein in the falciform ligament and in the liver.

1. diaphragm
2. intestine
3. kidney
4. liver
5. lung
6. pericardium
7. stomach
8. suprarenal (adrenal) gland
9. umbilical cord

160a. Week 10. The anterior (ventral) surface of the liver has been removed. 57 mm CR ♂

160b. Week 13. 101 mm CR ♀

161a–161d. Posterior (dorsal) surface of the liver.

161a. Week 10. 57 mm CR ♂

161b. Week 11. 65 mm CR ♂

161c. Week 13. 92 mm CR ♀

161d. Week 13. 101 mm CR ♀

162a. Stage 23 (Days 56–57). Transverse section of the liver. 29 mm CR

162b. Stage 23 (Days 56–57). Transverse section of the gallbladder. 30 mm CR

1. anterior abdominal wall	3. liver
2. gallbladder	4. stomach

1. bare area	5. gallbladder	9. porta hepatis
2. caudate lobe	6. gastric impression	10. quadrate lobe
3. colic impression	7. left lobe of liver	11. renal impression
4. esophageal groove	8. ligamentum teres and falciform ligament	12. right lobe of liver

Midgut rotation

In Week 4 the early intestine is a straight tube (see Yolk sac), but then in Weeks 5 and 6 it grows to form a single loop supplied centrally by the superior mesenteric artery. Two landmarks are present on the loop: the yolk stalk and the cecal diverticulum, which marks the join between the small and large intestine. The yolk stalk is at the apex of the loop dividing it into two parts: a cranial or proximal limb and a caudal or distal limb. The early abdomen (Week 6) is occupied primarily by the liver and kidneys; the rapidly growing intestine occupies an extra-embryonic position in the umbilical cord (physiological umbilical herniation). The proximal limb of the intestine grows very rapidly and forms several coils while the distal limb grows very slowly. As the opening into the umbilical cord is narrow, rotation occurs in the apex region. The yolk stalk connection to the intestine shrinks and breaks, the distal intestinal coil rotates 90° anticlockwise, so the cecal diverticulum (and distal limb) is carried toward the left-hand side of the body. The cecum and appendix are differentiating from the cecal diverticulum as the intestine returns (reduction) to the larger abdominal cavity (Week 10). The proximal limb of the intestine returns first (Week 8) and passes behind the superior mesenteric artery. The majority returns at Week 9. The returning large intestine rotates another 180° clockwise, so the appendix and cecum lie near the right lobe of the liver. Later, as they descend into the right iliac fossa, the proximal part of the colon forms the ascending colon and hepatic flexure.

As the intestines reach their adult positions, their mesenteries are pressed against the posterior abdominal wall where all the mesenteries are retained except that of the midgut duodenum and the ascending colon. The duodenum (except for the first 25 mm in the adult) and the ascending colon are retroperitoneal.

The proximal limb will form the 5.5–6.0 m of adult small intestine (duodenum, jejunum, and upper part of ileum). The distal limb, which will form the large intestine, is less in diameter than that of the small intestine until Week 18.

During Weeks 6–7 the epithelial lining of the duodenum proliferates and almost fills the lumen, but it is quickly re-established (Week 8).

Villi appear in Week 7, and the intestinal mucosa absorbs fluid from the amniotic fluid. The glands of Lieberkuhn appear at the base of the villi toward the end of Week 12 and Brunner's glands (duodenal) shortly afterward. Lymph nodes and Peyer's patches are present from Weeks 18–20. Elastic tissue is primarily in the blood vessel walls. The musculature is poorly developed and peristalsis is weak and discontinuous.

- Meckel's diverticulum is the persistence of the yolk stalk connection as an ileal diverticulum.
- The neonatal intestine is sterile at birth, but a bacterial flora is quickly acquired.
- The intestinal musculature is poorly developed at birth and the intestinal wall thin. In the first few months elastic tissue increases greatly in the walls.

163. Stage 17 (Day 41). The midgut is beginning to herniate into the umbilical cord. Viewed by transmitted light from the right side. 12 mm CR

1. arm bud
2. back
3. eye (right)
4. heart
5. leg bud
6. liver
7. midgut herniation
8. tail
9. umbilical cord

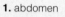

164. Stages 16–17 (Days 37–41). The midgut herniating into the umbilical cord. 12 mm CR

1. abdomen
2. arm bud (right)
3. genital tubercle
4. leg bud
5. midgut herniation
6. tail
7. umbilical cord

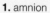

165. Stages 17–18 (Days 41–44). Midgut herniation. 14 mm CR

1. amnion
2. leg bud
3. midgut herniation
4. tail

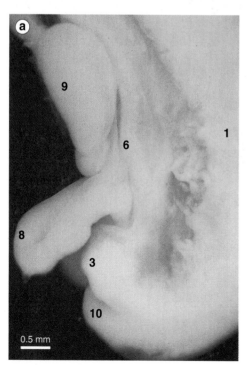

166a. Stages 17–18 (Days 41–44). Midgut herniation, viewed from the left side. The left leg bud and liver have been removed. 14 mm CR

166b. Same embryo as in **166a**, viewed from the right side. Note the dorsal mesentery in the loop of the midgut.

1. back
2. cactus needle
3. genital tubercle
4. leg bud
5. mesentery
6. mesonephric kidney (left)
7. midgut
8. midgut herniation (umbilical cord removed)
9. stomach
10. tail

167. Stage 18 (Day 44). Sagittal section illustrating midgut herniation. 16 mm CR

1. brain
2. genital tubercle
3. heart
4. liver
5. lung
6. mandible
7. midgut herniation
8. nose

1 mm

167 from CCHMS

168a–168c. Midgut herniation, viewed from the right.

1. abdomen
2. arm
3. elbow
4. finger
5. foot
6. knee
7. leg (right)
8. midgut herniation
9. rib
10. toe
11. umbilical cord

0.5 mm

168a. Stage 19 (Days 47–48). 20 mm CR

1 mm

168b. Stages 22–23 (Days 54–57). 27 mm CR

1 mm

168c. Week 8. 34 mm CR

169. Stages 22–23 (Days 54–57). Paraffin wax transverse section of the herniated midgut. 28 mm CR

1. aorta
2. erector spinae muscles
3. gonad
4. herniated midgut
5. kidney
6. liver
7. spinal cord
8. stomach
9. umbilical cord
10. vertebral body

169 from LHSM

170a and **170b.** The midgut herniation.

1. appendix
2. arm
3. esophagus
4. head
5. intestines
6. knee
7. leg
8. linea alba
9. stomach
10. umbilical cord

170a. Stages 22–23 (Days 54–57). The midgut herniation viewed from the front. 28 mm CR

170b. Week 8. Midgut herniation dissected from the umbilical cord. 40 mm CR

1 mm

1. abdomen
2. arm
3. ear
4. eye
5. leg
6. umbilical cord

5 mm

171. Week 11. Midgut herniation has returned to the enlarged abdominal cavity. 70 mm CR ♀

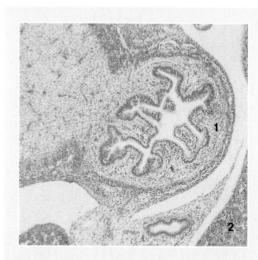

172. Stage 23 (Days 56–57). Transverse section of the duodenum. 30 mm CR

1. duodenum
2. liver

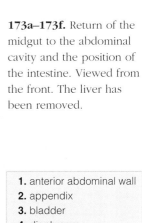

173a–173f. Return of the midgut to the abdominal cavity and the position of the intestine. Viewed from the front. The liver has been removed.

1. anterior abdominal wall
2. appendix
3. bladder
4. diaphragm
5. esophagus
6. gonad
7. greater omentum
8. herniated midgut
9. kidney
10. leg
11. stomach
12. suprarenal (adrenal) gland
13. transverse colon
14. umbilical cord

173a. Week 8. 34 mm CR

173b. Week 9. There is no difference in external appearance at this stage between small and large intestines. 50 mm CR ♀

173c. Week 11. 65 mm CR ♂

173d. Week 13. 97 mm CR ♂

173e. Week 15. 123 mm CR ♀

173f. Week 18. 152 mm CR ♂

1. anterior abdominal wall
2. diaphragm
3. esophagus
4. greater omentum
5. kidney
6. leg
7. site of hepatic flexure
8. stomach
9. suprarenal (adrenal) gland
10. transverse colon
11. umbilical cord

174a. Week 9. Intestinal villi. 50 mm CR

1. villi

174b. Week 10. Villi fill the intestine. 60 mm CR ♀

175. Full term fetus. Meckel's diverticulum (yolk sac stalk).

1. ilium
2. Meckel's diverticulum

175 from RFHSM

Hindgut

The midline hindgut is continuous with the caudal midgut and ends in the primitive cloaca (see Yolk sac). The allantois lies anterior to the anterior cloaca. In Weeks 6–7 the urorectal septum divides the cloaca and cloacal membrane into two parts, one comprising the rectum, anal canal, and anal membrane, and the other the urogenital sinus and urogenital membrane. The perineal body forms where the septum fuses with the cloacal membrane. Mesoderm proliferates around the anal membrane and causes the proctodeum (or anal pit) to form. In Week 8 the membrane ruptures and the anal canal communicates with the amniotic cavity.

The hindgut moves to the left as the midgut coils return to the abdominal cavity. It gives rise to the distal part of the transverse colon, the descending and sigmoid colon, the rectum, the upper part of the anal canal, and part of the urogenital system.

The inferior mesenteric artery supplies the hindgut.

The mesentery of the descending colon fuses with peritoneum on the left dorsal abdominal wall, and so disappears. The sigmoid colon's mesentery is retained.

The colon has poorly developed tenia coli and the external surface is smooth because it lacks haustra (sacculations) and appendices epiploicae. The colon contains the ingested amniotic fluid and sloughed skin epithelial cells, oral cavity cells, upper respiratory and intestinal tract cells, lanugo hairs, *vernix caseosa*, secretions of the liver, pancreas, and gastrointestinal glands, urea, steroids, biliverdin, mucoproteins, and mucopolysaccharides. Lipid is absorbed and the remaining contents collect in the colon as meconium after Weeks 16–20. At birth the rectum is usually distended with meconium.

- Haustra are formed during the first 6 months.
- Full-term infants defecate within 24 h of birth.

176a. Week 11. 65 mm CR ♂

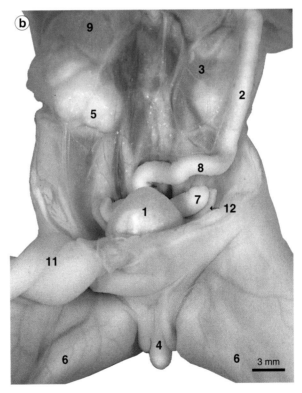

176b. Week 13. 92 mm CR ♀

176a–176e.
Development of the descending colon and rectum. In order not to obscure the view, the abdominal organs have been reflected cephalically (superiorly).

1. bladder
2. descending colon
3. descending mesocolon
4. external genitalia
5. kidney
6. leg
7. ovary
8. sigmoid colon
9. suprarenal (adrenal) gland
10. testis
11. umbilical cord
12. uterine (Fallopian) tube

176c. Week 13. 101 mm CR ♀

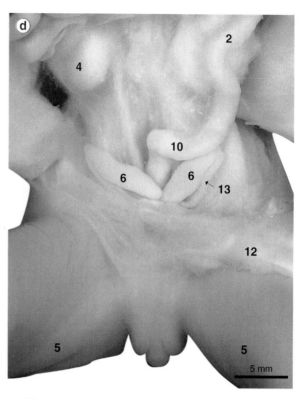

176d. Week 15. 123 mm CR ♀

1. bladder
2. descending colon
3. descending mesocolon
4. kidney
5. leg
6. ovary
7. penis
8. rectum (position)
9. scrotum
10. sigmoid colon
11. testis
12. umbilical cord
13. uterine (Fallopian) tube

176e. Week 18. 152 mm CR ♂

177. Week 15. The bladder and part of the uterovaginal primordium have been removed to display the position of the rectum in **176d.** 123 mm CR ♀

Cecum and vermiform appendix

The cecal diverticulum is present on the early intestine (Week 6) as a blunt area marking the joining of the small and large intestine. Later (Week 8) as the terminal part of the diverticulum (appendix) does not grow as rapidly as the proximal part (cecum), it forms a long blind sac. As the colon elongates the cecum and appendix descend, so that the appendix may lie posterior to the cecum (rectrocecal) or colon (retrocolic), or in a pelvic position.

- The appendix is relatively longer in the neonate in comparison with the adult.
- The cecum is relatively smaller in the neonate than in the adult.
- In the newborn, the cecum tapers into the appendix and there is usually no sharp demarcation between the two regions.
- In the neonate the haustra and appendices epiploicae are absent. The haustra develop in the first 6 months after birth.

178a. Stages 17–18 (Days 41–44). Early cecal diverticulum viewed from the left side. The umbilical cord has been removed. 14 mm CR

1. cecal diverticulum
2. heart
3. leg bud (left)
4. liver removed
5. mesonephric kidney
6. stomach
7. tail

178b. Stage 19 (Days 47–48). Cecal diverticulum viewed from the right side. The umbilical cord has been removed. 20 mm CR

1. abdomen
2. cactus needle
3. cecal diverticulum (with appendix)
4. midgut herniation (umbilical cord removed)

178c. Higher magnification of **178b.**

1 mm

0.5 mm

178d–178g. Further development of the cecum and appendix, viewed from the dorsal (back) surface.

178d. Week 9. 48 mm CR ♀

1. adrenal
2. appendix
3. intestine
4. kidney
5. liver
6. mesentery

178e. Week 10. 60 mm CR ♀

1 mm

178f. Week 10. 60 mm CR ♀

178g. Week 15. 123 mm CR ♀

2 mm

Anal canal

The anal canal has a dual origin: the upper two-thirds is from hindgut (supplied by the inferior mesenteric artery) and the lower third (supplied by the internal pudendal artery) is from proctodeum (see Hindgut). Approximately where the two join is marked by the pectinate line.

The anal sphincter musculature is well-developed at birth.

● If the fetus is anoxic, active peristalsis of the colon and rectum occurs and meconium enters the anal canal. The defecation reflex occurs, the anal sphincter muscles relax, and meconium passes into the amniotic fluid.

0.5 mm

179a–179h.
Development of the anus.

1. developing anus
2. external genitals
3. genital tubercle
4. leg
5. leg bud
6. tail
7. umbilical cord

179a. Stages 17–18 (Days 41–44). 14 mm CR

179b. Week 8. 32 mm CR

0.5 mm

179c. Week 8. 34 mm CR

0.5 mm

179d. Week 9. 48 mm CR

179e. Week 10. 56 mm CR ♀

179f. Week 12. 85 mm CR ♂

1. anus
2. buttocks
3. external genitals
4. leg
5. tail

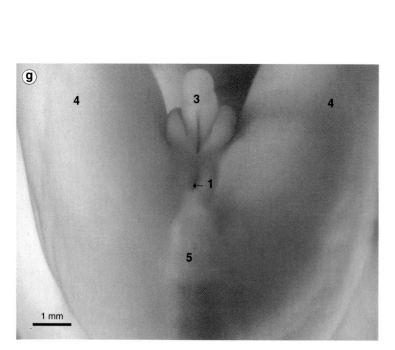

179g. Week 9. Relationship between the developing anus and the receding tail. 46 mm CR

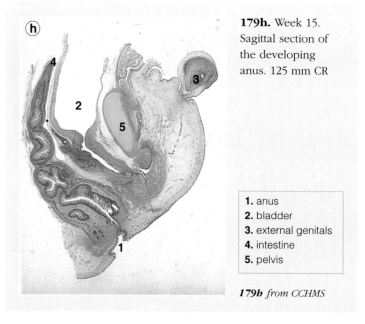

179h. Week 15. Sagittal section of the developing anus. 125 mm CR

1. anus
2. bladder
3. external genitals
4. intestine
5. pelvis

179b from CCHMS

Kidney

The lower cervical and upper thoracic intermediate mesoderm fuse to form a continuous nephrogenic cord. At Days 23–24 the primary excretory duct forms in the dorsal nephrogenic cord at the ninth somite level and as it grows caudally, it separates from the nephrogenic cord and becomes hollow. It lies immediately below the ectoderm and turns ventrally to open into the cloaca at Day 28. A diverticulum, the metanephric or ureteric bud, is found where the cord enters the cloaca.

Clusters of cells in the cranial nephrogenic cord form rudimentary and transient nephric tubules: the pronephroi.

The mesonephroi succeed the pronephroi and form caudally at the L3 level. At one end, the 'S' shaped mesonephric tubules open into the primary excretory duct (now the mesonephric duct), and at the other end is found a glomerular capsule with a vascular supply from the aorta. The more cranial tubules atrophy and disappear before the more caudal ones develop. Usually, no more than 30–40 tubules are present at one time in an embryo. By the end of Week 6 the mesonephroi together form the mesonephric ridge which is present from the septum transversum to the L3 level. The genital gland forms on its medial aspect. Most of the cranial mesonephroi atrophy and disappear until only those at the L1–L3 level remain.

Derivatives of the remaining tubules are the efferent ductules of the testis and paradidymis in the male and the epoophoron and paroophoron in the female.

In the male, the mesonephric duct forms the appendix of the epididymis, vas (ductus) deferens, and ejaculatory duct. At the end of Week 13 the seminal vesicle and ampulla of the ductus deferens form at the end of the mesonephric duct. At Week 15 the two areas separate and at Week 24 development of the mesonephric duct is suppressed and both areas grow rapidly.

In the female, development of the mesonephric duct is suppressed and it forms the longitudinal duct of the epoophoron, appendix vesiculosa, and duct of Gartner.

As the metanephric (ureteric) bud grows dorsally from the mesonephric duct in Week 5, its blind end grows into a mass of metanephric mesoderm which forms the metanephric cap. The stalk of the ureteric bud forms the ureter, and gives rise to the pelvis, calyces, and collecting tubules. Derivatives of the metanephric cap are the nephrons. Glomerular blood vessels form *in situ*. Urine is formed at Week 9 and is excreted into the amniotic fluid (see Amnion).

Blood supply

The pelvic kidney is supplied by the common iliac arteries. As the kidney migrates cephalically, it is supplied successively by new aortic branches. Finally, at Week 9 it is supplied by the most caudal suprarenal artery (from the aorta) which enlarges to form the renal artery.

- The neonatal kidney is lobulated, but the lobulation is usually lost by 4–5 years of age.
- The glomeruli become fully functional about 6 weeks after birth.
- The absence of one kidney (renal agenesis) is relatively common.
- Kidneys containing multiple cysts (polycystic) function poorly. The exact cause of the cysts is uncertain.

180a–180l. Development of the mesonephric and metanephric kidneys.

180a. Stages 17–18 (Days 41–44). Viewed from the ventral surface. The mesonephric kidney is running the length of the abdomen. The liver has been removed. 14 mm CR

180b. Same specimen as in **180a**, viewed from the ventral surface. The stomach has been reflected to the right side.

180c. View from the left side of the embryo in **180a**.

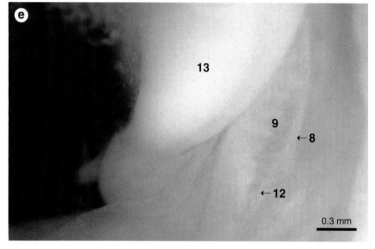

180d. View from the left side of the embryo in **180a**.

180e. Higher magnification of **180d**.

1. abdomen
2. back
3. cactus needle
4. heart
5. leg bud
6. liver
7. lung bud
8. mesonephric duct
9. mesonephric tubules
10. metanephric bud
11. midgut
12. paramesonephric duct
13. stomach
14. tail

180f. View from the right side of the embryo in **180a**.

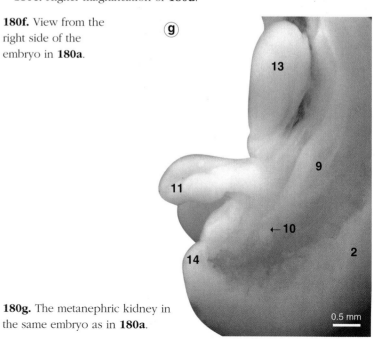

180g. The metanephric kidney in the same embryo as in **180a**.

180j–180l. The metanephric kidney.

180j. Week 8. The intestine has been reflected superiorly. 40 mm CR

180k. Week 8. 48 mm CR ♀

180h. Stage 19 (Days 47–48). The mesonephric kidney degenerating as the metanephric kidney migrates up the posterior abdominal wall to meet the suprarenal (adrenal) gland. Liver removed, viewed from the left. 20 mm CR

1. gonad
2. mesonephric kidney
3. mesonephric tubules
4. metanephric kidney
5. midgut
6. pancreas
7. suprarenal (adrenal) gland

180i. Same specimen as in **180h**.

180l. Week 10. 56 mm CR

1. bladder
2. gonad
3. intestine (and appendix)
4. kidney (metanephric)
5. leg
6. liver
7. suprarenal (adrenal) gland

181. Week 18. Final position of the fetal kidney. 152 mm CR ♂

1. back
2. diaphragm
3. fat
4. intestine
5. kidney

10 mm

a
b
c
d

0.5 mm

5 mm

5 mm

5 mm

182a–182d. Increase in size of the metanephric kidney and the suprarenal (adrenal) gland.

182a. Week 9. View of the ventral surface. 48 mm CR ♂

182b. Week 11. 65 mm CR ♂

182c. Week 13. 101 mm CR ♀

182d. Week 18. Left kidney and suprarenal gland. View of the dorsal surface. 152 mm CR ♂

1. metanephric kidney
2. suprarenal (adrenal) gland
3. ureter

183a–183c. Transverse paraffin wax sections of the mesonephroi in the early embryo.

183a. Stages 15–16 (Days 33–37). 8 mm CR   *183a from LHSM*

183b. Stages 15–16 (Days 33–37). 9 mm CR

183c. Higher magnification of the mesonephric tubules in **183b**.

1. dorsal aortae
2. gonadal ridge
3. hindgut
4. intraembryonic coelom
5. mesonephric glomerulus
6. mesonephric ridge

184a–184g. Transverse paraffin wax sections of metanephric kidney development.

184a. Stages 22–23 (Days 54–57). 28 mm CR

184c. Week 8. 40 mm CR   *184c from St T*

184b. Week 8. 35 mm CR

184b from Mr G. Bottomley

184d. Week 10. 60 mm CR ♀

1. aorta	**4.** glomeruli	**7.** major calyx	**10.** minor calyx	**13.** ureter
2. cortex	**5.** gonad	**8.** medulla	**11.** spinal cord	**14.** vertebral body
3. erector spinae muscles	**6.** kidney	**9.** mesonephroi	**12.** suprarenal gland	

1. collecting tubules
2. cortex
3. glomeruli
4. kidney
5. medulla

184e. Week 14. *184e from QUB*
105 mm CR

184g. Week 19. 170 mm CR   *184g from QUB*

184f. Week 18. 152 mm CR ♂

1. abdominal
   wall
2. bladder
   wall
3. colon
4. fat
5. gonad
6. kidney
7. umbilical
   artery
8. umbilical
   cord
9. urachus
10. ureter

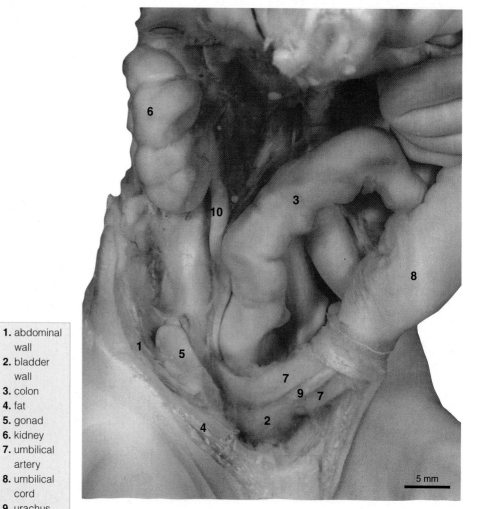

185. Week 18. Relative positions of the ureter, kidney, and bladder.
152 mm CR ♂

5 mm

RELATIVE POSITION OF THE KIDNEY

The kidneys form in the pelvic cavity early in Week 5 and migrate cranially onto the posterior abdominal wall. At Days 34–36 they have reached the level of L2. The renal pelvis, which originally faces ventrally rotates to a medial position.

In Week 9, the kidneys rise to meet the suprarenal (adrenal) glands on the posterior abdominal wall.

186a and **186b.** Mesonephric and metanephric kidneys in the early embryo, viewed from the left.

186a. Stages 17–18 (Days 41–44) 14 mm CR

186b. Stage 19 (Days 47–48). 20 mm CR

1. back
2. genital tubercle
3. gonad
4. intestine
5. mesonephric kidney
6. metanephric kidney
7. pancreas
8. stomach
9. suprarenal (adrenal) gland
10. umbilical cord

0.5 mm

187a–187f. Relative positions of the developing kidney, viewed from the front.

1. bladder
2. external genitals
3. gonads
4. intestine
5. kidney
6. leg
7. suprarenal (adrenal) gland
8. umbilical cord

1 mm

1 mm

2 mm

187a. Week 8. 40 mm CR ♀

187b. Week 9. 50 mm CR ♀

187c. Week 9. 50 mm CR ♀

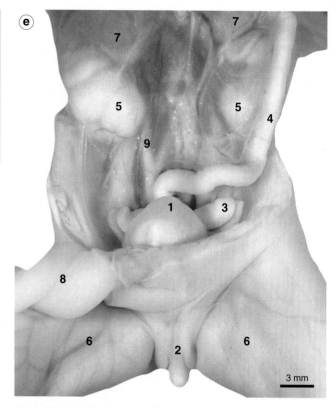

1. bladder
2. external genitals
3. gonads
4. intestine
5. kidney
6. leg
7. suprarenal
   (adrenal) gland
8. umbilical cord
9. ureter

187d. Week 9. 57 mm CR ♀

187e. Week 13. 92 mm CR ♀

187f. Week 15. 123 mm CR ♀

187g. Week 18. Dorsal (back) view of the final position of the kidneys. The ribs have been reflected forward. 152 mm CR ♂

1. diaphragm   4. lung
2. fat   5. ribs
3. kidney   6. suprarenal gland

Suprarenal (adrenal) glands

The suprarenal has a dual origin: the medulla from neural crest cells and the cortex from mesoderm.

The fetal cortex appears in Week 6 when cells from the coelomic epithelium aggregate on each side between the developing gonad and the dorsal mesentery. The medullary cells migrate from adjacent sympathetic ganglia (neural crest) and form a mass on the medial surface of the fetal cortex. Gradually, the medullar mass, which forms the chromaffin cells, is surrounded by the fetal cortex. A second layer of investing mesoderm forms the adult cortex.

Between Weeks 8 and 9 the cortex produces corticosteroids. The cortex also produces androgens and estriol precursors.

The medulla produces insignificant quantities of epinephrine (adrenalin).

- The neonatal gland is 20 times the relative size of the gland in the adult.
- The zona glomerulosa and the zona fasciculata are present in the neonatal suprarenal.
- The fetal cortex disappears by the age of one year and the suprarenal rapidly becomes absolutely smaller.
- The zona reticularis forms by the end of the third year.

188a–188g. Development of the suprarenal (adrenal) gland. (Also see Kidney.)

188a. Stage 19 (Days 47–48). Early suprarenal gland, viewed from the right side. The liver has been removed. 20 mm CR

1. gonad
2. kidney (metanephric)
3. mesonephric kidney
4. suprarenal gland

188b. Week 8. View from the ventral surface. 40 mm CR

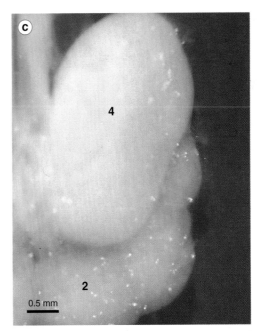

188c. Higher magnification of the suprarenal gland in **188b**.

d

188d. Week 10. View of the ventral surface. 56 mm CR

1 mm

e

188e. Week 10. View of the ventral surface. 60 mm CR ♀

1 mm

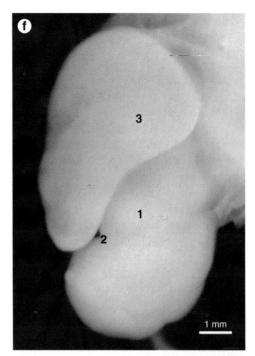

f

188f. Week 11. View from the ventral surface. 65 mm CR ♂

1 mm

g

188g. Dorsal view of the specimen in **188f**.

1 mm

1. kidney
2. pelvis of kidney
3. suprarenal gland

189. Stage 23 (Days 56–57). A transverse section of the suprarenal gland. 30 mm CR

1. liver
2. suprarenal gland

Urinary bladder

The urorectal septum divides the cloaca into the urogenital sinus and the rectum and anal canal. The allantois is continuous with and ends in the urogenital sinus. The mesonephric ducts also end in the urogenital sinus. The bladder forms from the cranial part of the urogenital sinus. As the bladder enlarges, the mesonephric ducts (the ductus deferens in the male) and ureter are incorporated into the dorsal wall so that they enter the bladder separately. The mesonephric ducts contribute to the trigone of the bladder, but their mesodermal epithelium is soon replaced by urogenital sinus endodermal epithelium. In the female, the caudal ends of the mesonephric ducts subsequently degenerate. The surrounding splanchnic mesoderm forms the other layers of the bladder.

As the bladder grows, the allantois forms the tubular urachus, which then becomes a fibrous cord passing from the apex of the bladder to the umbilicus. This cord is the median umbilical ligament.

FEMALE URETHRA

The epithelium is derived from the endodermal urogenital sinus. Adjacent splanchnic mesoderm forms the connective tissue and smooth muscle.

MALE URETHRA

The epithelium is derived from the urogenital sinus (except the glandular part of the penile urethra). The connective tissue and smooth muscle are from adjacent splanchnic mesoderm. The epithelium of the cranial prostatic part is mesodermal originally, but is replaced by endodermal epithelium.

The glandular penile urethra forms by an ectodermal ingrowth at the tip of the penis splitting to form a urethral groove.

- There is no true fundus in the neonatal bladder.
- The bladder contains a small amount of urine at birth.
- The fully distended bladder in the young infant is almost entirely abdominal and may extend up to the umbilicus.
- Hypospadias in the male is failure or incomplete fusion of the urogenital folds, and results in an incomplete penile urethra.

190a–190f. The bladder.

190a. Stage 19 (Days 47–48). View from the right. 20 mm CR

190b. Week 9. The umbilical cord has been pulled taut. View from the front of the rostral surface. 48 mm CR

190c. Week 10. The caudal surface of the bladder, viewed from below. The legs have been removed. 56 mm CR

1. allantois
2. buttocks
3. cactus needle
4. early bladder
5. external genitals
6. intestine
7. leg
8. umbilical arteries
9. umbilical cord

190d. Week 11. Rostral surface, viewed from the front. 65 mm CR ♂

190e. Caudal surface of the same specimen in **190d**, viewed from below.

1. anterior abdominal wall
2. bladder
3. clitoris
4. intestine
5. kidney
6. leg
7. ovary
8. penis
9. testis
10. umbilical artery
11. umbilical cord

190f. Week 13. Caudal surface, viewed from the front. 92 mm CR ♀

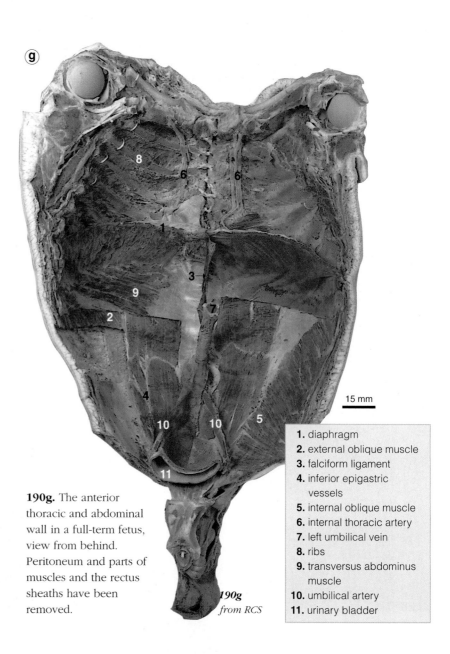

190g. The anterior thoracic and abdominal wall in a full-term fetus, view from behind. Peritoneum and parts of muscles and the rectus sheaths have been removed.

190g from RCS

1. diaphragm
2. external oblique muscle
3. falciform ligament
4. inferior epigastric vessels
5. internal oblique muscle
6. internal thoracic artery
7. left umbilical vein
8. ribs
9. transversus abdominus muscle
10. umbilical artery
11. urinary bladder

191. Week 9. Transverse section through the bladder and urethra. 49 mm CR

191 from CCHMS

1. bladder	5. rectum
2. femur	6. spinal cord
3. labioscrotal swelling	7. urethra
4. phallus	8. vertebral body

192a–192c. The developing bladder, viewed in sagittal section.

1. bladder
2. penis
3. rectum
4. scrotum
5. urethra
6. vertebral column

192d. Full-term fetus. Sagittal section through the bladder and urethra. A red bristle has been inserted in the urethra. Note the fetal position of the bladder.

192d from RFHSM

193a–193e. Development of the genital tubercle, viewed from the right side.

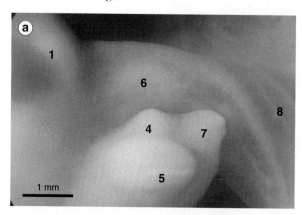

193a. Stages 16–17 (Days 37–41). 12 mm CR

193b. Stages 16–17 (Days 37–41). 12 mm CR

193c. Stages 17–18 (Days 41–44). 14 mm CR

193d. Stage 19 (Days 47–48). 20 mm CR

193e. Stage 19 (Days 47–48). 20 mm CR

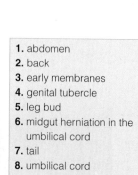

1. abdomen
2. back
3. early membranes
4. genital tubercle
5. leg bud
6. midgut herniation in the umbilical cord
7. tail
8. umbilical cord

Genitals: external

INDIFFERENT STAGE

Until Week 9 the external genitalia of the two sexes are similar in appearance.

Initially, a midline genital tubercle is present cephalic to the proctodeal depression (Week 4). This tubercle will form the penis or clitoris. At the caudal surface of the genital tubercle are two labioscrotal swellings enclosing two urogenital folds which enclose the cloacal membrane. The genital tubercle elongates to form a phallus* and is as big in the female as in the male. As the tubercle elongates it carries a projection from the urogenital sinus (urethral groove). At Week 6 the urorectal septum fuses with the cloacal membrane dividing it into a ventral urogenital membrane and a dorsal anal membrane. Shortly after Week 6 the urogenital membrane breaks down and the urethral groove and urogenital orifice are continuous.

* The term 'phallus' is used to denote the indifferent stage of development.

194a and **194b.** Week 9. Formation of the phallus, viewed from below. 48 mm CR

1. anus
2. labioscrotal swelling
3. phallus
4. urethral groove continuous with the urogenital sinus
5. urogenital folds

194a. Unfused urogenital folds

194b. Urethral groove continuous with the urogenital sinus, viewed by transmitted light.

194c. Week 9. Relationship between the anus, genitals, and tail. 48 mm CR

1. anus
2. back (dorsal) surface
3. labioscrotal swelling
4. leg
5. phallus
6. tail
7. urethral groove continuous with the urogenital sinus

195. Clitoris of a
female fetus, view
from the side.
Note the epithelial
tag. 43 mm CR

0.5 mm

1. clitoris
2. epithelial tag
3. leg

FEMALE

The genital tubercle forms the phallus, which develops into the clitoris (Week 9). The urogenital folds do not fuse (except immediately in front of the anus) and form the labia minora. The labioscrotal swellings do not fuse (except cephalically to form the anterior labial commissure and the mons pubis, and caudally to form the posterior labial commissure) and form the labia majora (Weeks 9–12). The labia majora are homologous with the male scrotum.

A primitive urethral groove forms but regresses. The female urethra is homologous to the upper portion of the prostatic part of the male urethra (see Male urethra).

196a and **196b.** Development of the female external genitalia, view from below.

0.5 mm

1. anus
2. buttock
3. clitoris
4. labioscrotal swelling (labia majora)
5. leg
6. urogenital fold (labia minora)

196a. Week 9. 46 mm CR

196b. Week 12. 85 mm CR

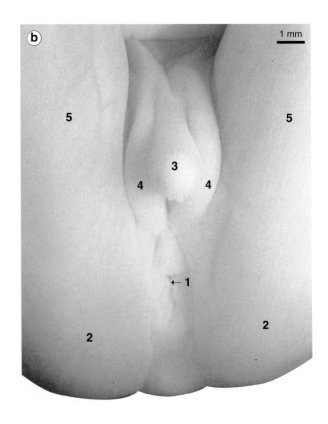

1 mm

197a–197f. Development of the female external genitalia, view from below.

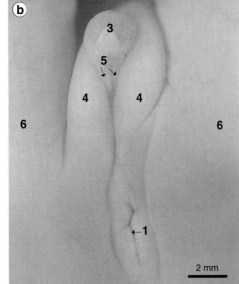

1. anus
2. buttock
3. clitoris
4. labia majora
5. labia minora
6. leg
7. meconium

197a. Week 13. 92 mm CR

197b. Week 13. 101 mm CR

197c. Week 15. 130 mm CR

197d. Week 17. 150 mm CR

197e. Week 20. 185 mm CR

197f. Week 35.

198. Neonatal external genitalia. A complete hymen is present. Note the small development of the labia minora.

198 from RFHSM

1. anus
2. clitoris
3. hymen
4. labia majora
5. labia minora

199a–199g. Male external genitalia, view from below.

199a. Week 9. The urogenital folds have started to fuse. 48 mm CR

1. anus	
2. labioscrotal swelling	
3. leg	
4. penis (glans)	
5. scrotal raphe	
6. scrotum	
7. urethral groove	
8. urogenital folds	

MALE

The genital tubercle elongates to form the phallus which develops into the penis. An epithelial tag is frequently attached to the tip of the phallus. On either side of the urethral groove are the urogenital folds.

At Week 9 the urogenital folds fuse from the posterior toward the tip. This produces a median penile raphe over the tubular urethra. The penile urethra forms when an ectodermal ingrowth at the tip of the glans splits to form a urethral groove. This is continuous with the urethral groove of the body (see Male urethra).

The prepuce forms at Week 12 as an epithelial fold which ingrows from the tip. Later (after birth), this fold splits to form the inner epithelial lining of the prepuce and the outer epithelial lining of the glans, so creating the preputial space between them.

The genital (labioscrotal) swellings fuse in the midline to form the scrotal raphe which is continuous with the perineal raphe. The corpora cavernosa and corpus spongiosum of the penis form from mesoderm in the phallus.

- Hypospadias results from incomplete fusion of the urogenital folds.
- The neonatal prepuce and glans may not be separated completely.

199b. Week 9. The urogenital folds have fused, except near the tip. 48 mm CR

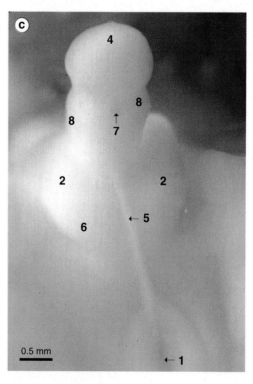

199c. Week 10. The urogenital folds have almost completely fused. 56 mm CR

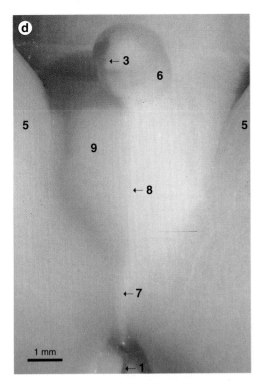

199d. Week 12. The urogenital folds have fused. Note the epithelial tag. 85 mm CR

199e. Week 13. The urethra is present at the top. 97 mm CR

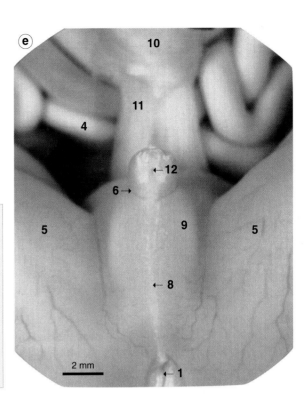

1. anus
2. buttocks
3. epithelial tag
4. intestines
5. leg
6. penis (body)
7. perineal raphe
8. scrotal raphe
9. scrotum
10. umbilical cord
11. urachus and umbilical arteries
12. urethra

199f. Week 18. The testes are not present in the scrotum. 160 mm CR

199g. Full-term fetus. The testes are present in the scrotum.

199g from RFHSM

199h. Transverse section of glans penis and prepuce. 300 mm CR

1. glans penis
2. prepuce

*199b from
J.D. Boyd Collection*

Gonads: internal

INDIFFERENT STAGE

Until Week 7 both sexes appear similar, even though their sex is determined at fertilization. The early period is the 'indifferent' stage of development.

Early in Week 4 primordial germ cells from the yolk sac migrate to the gonadal ridges which have developed on the medial side of the mesonephroi. Coelomic epithelial cords (primary sex cords) grow into the mesoderm of the gonadal ridge to produce an outer cortex and inner medulla.

During Week 6 the germ cells become incorporated into the gonad. In the female the medulla regresses, while in the male the cortex regresses and the medulla forms the testis.

Ducts

Two pairs of ducts form in both sexes: the mesonephric ducts (Wolffian) (see Kidney) and the paramesonephric (Müllerian) ducts. The latter form from coelomic epithelium and lie lateral and generally parallel to the mesonephric ducts. Their cranial ends open into the coelomic cavity and the caudal ends cross ventral to the mesonephric ducts and fuse in the midline to form a 'Y' shaped uterovaginal primordium in the female, which projects into the urogenital sinus. In the male, development of the paramesonephric duct is suppressed and the duct forms the appendix of the testis. The Müllerian tubercle is produced where the primordium enters the sinus. The tubercle will form the hymen in females and the seminal colliculus in males. The mesonephric ducts enter the sinus on either side of this tubercle.

200. Stages 15–16 (Days 33–37). Transverse paraffin wax section of the gonadal ridge. 8 mm CR   *200 from LHSM*

1. body wall	**4.** mesonephric glomeruli
2. dorsal aorta	**5.** notochord
3. gonadal ridge	

201a–201b. Stages 17–18 (Days 41–44). The gonadal ridge.

1. esophagus
2. gonadal ridge
3. mesonephric duct
4. mesonephric kidney
5. mesonephric tubules
6. midgut herniation (the umbilical cord has been removed)
7. paramesonephric duct
8. stomach

201a. View from the right side. The liver has been removed. 14 mm CR

201b. View from the left side.

FEMALE

Ovary

The formation of the early ovary is similar to that of the testis (see later), although the sex cords become broken up into isolated follicles and the tunica albuginea and rete are poorly developed.

Descent of the ovary

During Week 12 the ovary descends to a point below the pelvic brim. The middle part of the gubernaculum fuses with the body of the uterus dividing the gubernaculum into two parts: the upper part becomes the ovarian ligament and the lower part the round ligament of the uterus. The round ligament passes through the inguinal canal to end in the labium majus. A vaginal process forms, but disappears before birth. Estrogen secretion by the fetal ovaries is insignificant.

Uterus and vagina

The fused paramesonephric ducts form the uterovaginal primordium. This forms the epithelium and glands of the body and cervix of the uterus, and can be distinguished in Week 10. The cervix is longer than the body. The myometrium and endometrial stroma form from adjacent mesoderm. The unfused parts of the paramesonephric ducts form the uterine (Fallopian) tubes, whose open ends develop fimbria. The gubernaculum forms as the mesonephroi degenerates.

The uterovaginal region of the fused paramesonephric ducts expands to form the vaginal walls and canalization forms the vaginal lumen. Dilatation of the cephalic end produces the fornices. The caudal end expands and increases the area of contact with the urogenital sinus. The vaginal plate forms from the sinovaginal bulbs and forms the hymen which is placed superficially at birth.

- In the first weeks after birth, the uterus is no longer influenced by maternal hormones and involutes markedly.
- After birth, the ovaries assume their adult position on the posterior surface of the broad ligament.

202a and **202b.** Week 8. Urogenital organs of a female fetus dissected out. 40 mm CR

202a. View from the ventral side.

1. bladder
2. kidney
3. ovary
4. rectum
5. round ligament of the uterus
6. suprarenal (adrenal) gland
7. uterine tube
8. uterovaginal primordium

202b. Higher magnification of the organs in **202a**.

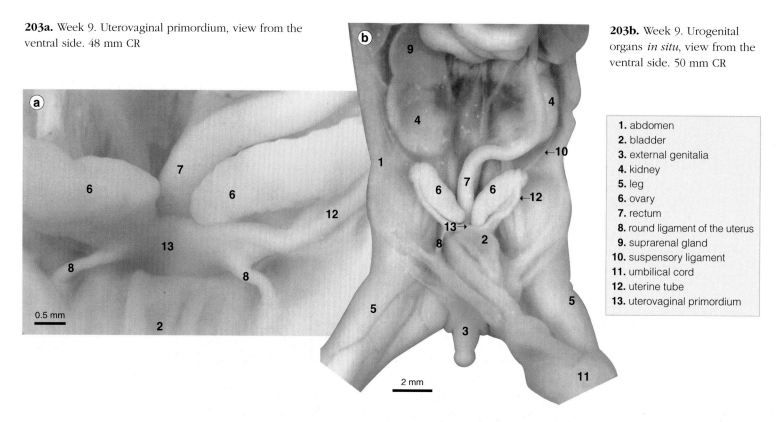

203a. Week 9. Uterovaginal primordium, view from the ventral side. 48 mm CR

0.5 mm

203b. Week 9. Urogenital organs *in situ*, view from the ventral side. 50 mm CR

2 mm

1. abdomen
2. bladder
3. external genitalia
4. kidney
5. leg
6. ovary
7. rectum
8. round ligament of the uterus
9. suprarenal gland
10. suspensory ligament
11. umbilical cord
12. uterine tube
13. uterovaginal primordium

204a and **204b.** Week 15. Course of the round ligament of the uterus, viewed from the ventral surface.

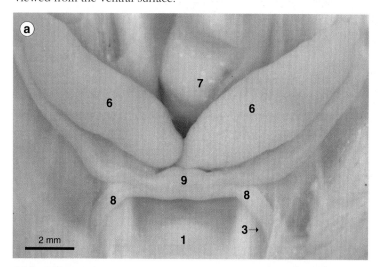

2 mm

204a. 123 mm CR

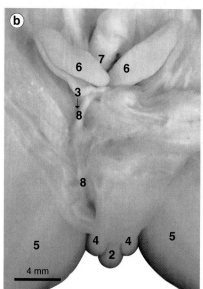

4 mm

204b. Same fetus as in **204a**.

1. bladder
2. clitoris
3. vaginal process
4. labia majora
5. leg
6. ovary
7. rectum
8. round ligament of the uterus
9. uterovaginal primordium

205. Week 13. Female internal genitalia dissected as a single tract. The lower uterus and vagina have been opened to illustrate the internal structure. 101 mm CR

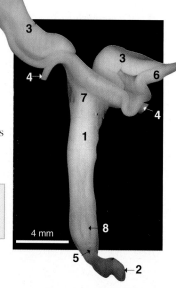

4 mm

1. body of the uterus
2. clitoris
3. ovary
4. round ligament of the uterus
5. solid epithelial plug where the vagina meets the urogenital sinus
6. uterine tube
7. uterus
8. vagina

MALE

Testis

In the male, the primary sex cords extend into the medulla where they branch, hollow out, and their ends anastomose to form the rete testis. The sex cords (seminiferous or testicular cords) lose their connection with the germinal epithelium as the connective tissue coat (tunica albuginea) forms. As the mesonephroi regress caudally, the testis separates and is suspended by its own mesentery, the mesorchium.

The seminiferous cords form the seminiferous tubules, rete testis, and tubuli recti. The walls of the seminiferous tubules are composed of two types of cells: supporting Sertoli cells, derived from germinal epithelium, and spermatogonia, derived from primordial germ cells. The seminiferous tubules become separated by Leydig cells (mesoderm).

The cephalic end of the mesonephric duct forms the appendix of the epididymis. The mesonephric duct also forms the duct of the epididymis, the ductus (vas) deferens and the ejaculatory duct. Where it enters the urogenital sinus, the ampulla of the vas deferens forms and a diverticulum from the ampulla forms the seminal vesicles. The caudal tubules of the mosonephroi form the paradidymis.

The paramesonephric duct disappears, except the cranial tip, which forms the appendix of the testis, and the caudal end which forms utriculus masculinus.

206a–206b. Development of the testis, view from the ventral surface.

1. anterior abdominal wall
2. bladder
3. buttock
4. leg
5. rectum
6. scrotum
7. testis
8. umbilical arteries
9. umbilical cord

206a. Week 13. 97 mm CR

206b. Week 13. The bladder and urachus have been lowered. 97 mm CR

207a and **207b.** Transverse paraffin wax sections of developing testis and prostate gland.

207a. Week 24. Testis.

207b.
Week 24.
Prostate
gland.

207a and 207b from QUB

Descent of the testis

As the mosonephroi degenerates the gubernaculum forms on the lower side of the testis, passes obliquely through the abdominal wall, and attaches to the scrotal swelling. The processus vaginalis, a sac of peritoneum carrying layers of the abdominal wall before it, forms ventral to the gubernaculum. These layers form the walls of the inguinal canal and the coverings of the spermatic cord and testis.

By Week 28 the testis, originally on the dorsal abdominal wall, has moved to the deep inguinal ring. The fetal body then elongates while the gubernaculum grows at a slower rate, so that the testis descends into the scrotum (Week 32).

Prostate gland

The prostate has a dual origin: the glandular epithelium forms from the numerous outgrowths of the prostatic urethral endoderm, and the stroma and smooth muscle form from surrounding mesoderm.

Bulbourethral gland

These glands have a dual origin: one part is an endodermal outgrowth of the spongy urethra, and another part is stroma and smooth muscle from the surrounding mesoderm.

● Sometimes the testes are undescended at birth, but descend into the scrotum during the first 3 months thereafter.

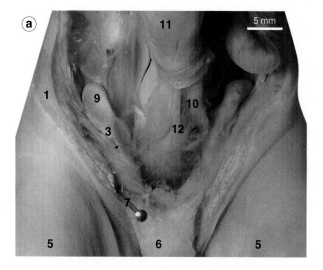

208a–208c Descent of the testis into the scrotum.

208a. Week 18. Testis in the abdominal cavity, viewed from the ventral surface. 152 mm CR

1. anterior abdominal wall
2. fat
3. inguinal canal
4. intestine
5. leg
6. penis
7. pin
8. scrotum
9. testis
10. umbilical artery
11. umbilical cord
12. urachus

*208b and 208c are in reverse age order because the fetus in 208b is less mature than that in 208c.

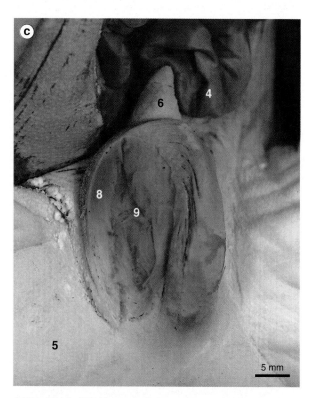

208b. Week 24*. Testis in the inguinal canal, view from the ventral surface. 228 mm CR

208c. Week 23*. Testis in the scrotum, view from below. 220 mm CR

Tail Formation

209a–209g. Regression and disappearance of the tail.

209a. Stage 17 (Day 41). View from the ventral surface. 12 mm CR

The human tail develops from the posterior body fold or tail fold. It normally reaches a maximum length of one-tenth that of the embryo during Week 5, and then disappears during the next 3–4 weeks by regression, cell death, and by the rapid increase in size of the buttock region. By term, the tail has developed into the coccygeal region.

● Very rarely a tail may be present at birth.

209b. Stages 17–18 (Days 41–44). View from the right side. 14 mm CR

209c. Stage 19 (Days 47–48). View from the back. 18 mm CR

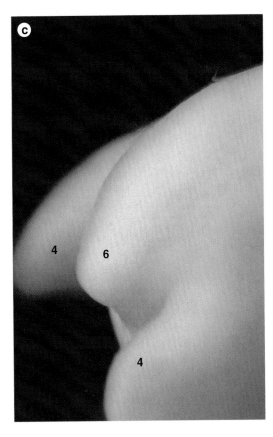

1. genitals
2. head
3. heart
4. leg bud
5. liver
6. tail
7. umbilical cord

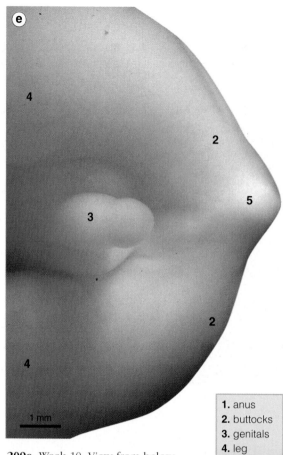

209d. Week 10. View from the right side.
57 mm CR ♂

209e. Week 10. View from below.
60 mm CR ♀

1. anus
2. buttocks
3. genitals
4. leg
5. tail

209f. Week 12. View from below.
85 mm CR ♂

209g. Week 13. View from below.
97 mm CR ♂

Limbs

The upper and lower limbs develop from buds of mesoderm covered by a layer of ectoderm. The upper limb first appears late in Week 4, followed 2 days later by the lower limb. This cephalo–caudal maturity gradient is retained throughout development.

ARM DEVELOPMENT AND ROTATION

The upper limb bud projects 90° from the body. The cranial border is called the preaxial border and the caudal border the postaxial. An apical ectodermal ridge influences development and growth of the limb. As the arm, forearm, and hand regions form (Week 5), the hand faces the trunk. At Weeks 7–9, the elbow is moved 90° dorsally.

HAND AND FOOT DEVELOPMENT

In Week 6 the upper limb bud develops a hand plate (paddle) distally, which is composed of digital (finger) rays separated by grooves. In Week 7 the lower limb bud foot plate has digital (toe) rays. Soon tissue in the grooves breaks down, and fingers or toes are produced in Week 8.

FINGERNAILS AND TOENAILS

During Week 10 the fingernails appear, followed by the toenails 4 weeks later. The ectoderm covering the dorsal aspect of the tip of each digit thickens to form a nail field. As the nail field grows it moves onto the dorsal surface, but because of its slow growth rate it becomes depressed, with the surrounding epidermis forming nail folds by overlapping the proximal and lateral parts of the nail field. The proximal part of the nail field becomes the formative zone, whose cells grow over the nail field, keratinize, and form the nail plate.

At first a thin layer of epidermis, the eponychium, covers the developing nail. Later, this degenerates, except for the cuticle.

The nails reach the fingertips by Week 32 and toetips by Week 36.

NERVE SUPPLY

Spinal nerves enter the brachial plexus from the cervical enlargement of the spinal cord. The plexus divides into anterior and posterior divisions which supply the flexor and extensor compartments respectively.

- Nails not reaching the finger- or toe-tips by birth, indicates prematurity.
- Infants are often born with faces scratched by their fingernails. It may be necessary to clip the nails at birth to prevent damage to the skin and eyes.

210a–210k. Development and rotation of the arm.

210a. Stages 14–15 (Days 32–33). Coronal section of the early arm bud. 7 mm CR

210a from LHSM

210b. Stages 15–16 (Days 33–37). Arm bud sectioned coronally. 10 mm CR

1. apical ectodermal ridge
2. arm bud
3. cervical and thoracic spinal nerves
4. dorsal surface
5. postaxial border
6. preaxial border
7. somites

210c. Stages 13–14 (Days 28–32). Arm bud, viewed from behind.

210d. Stages 16–18 (Days 37–44). Arm bud. 14 mm CR

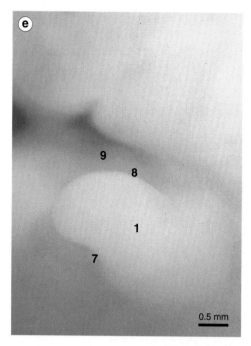

210e. Stages 16–18 (Days 37–44). The arm bud has turned medially. 14 mm CR

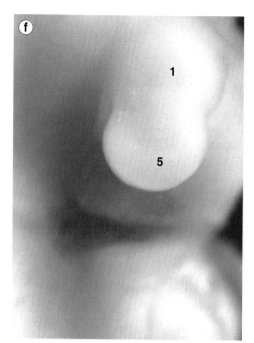

210f. Stages 16–17 (Days 37–41). The hand plate is present. 14 mm CR

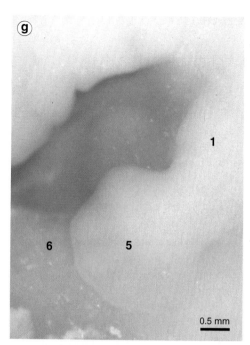

210g. Stage 17 (Day 41). The hand plate is present. Note the future thumb is recognizable. The younger specimen is more mature than the embryo in **210e** and **210f**. 12 mm CR

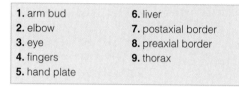

1. arm bud	**6.** liver
2. elbow	**7.** postaxial border
3. eye	**8.** preaxial border
4. fingers	**9.** thorax
5. hand plate	

210h. Stage 22 (Day 54). The arm has bent at the elbow, which points caudally. The arm moves *in utero* from Weeks 7–8. 27 mm CR

210i. Stage 22 (Day 54). The hands meet and cross in the midline over the thorax. 27 mm CR

1. elbow
2. eye
3. fingers
4. postaxial border
5. preaxial border
6. thorax
7. umbilical cord

210j. Week 13. 97 mm CR ♂

210k. Week 18. 152 mm CR ♂

211. Week 20. Ultrasound scan of limbs.

1. arm
2. back
3. head
4. leg

211 from Mr P. Baines

212a–212j. Hand and finger development.

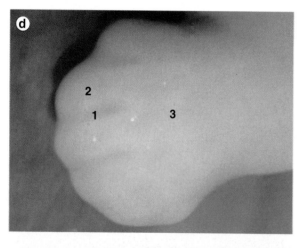

212a. Stages 16–17 (Days 37–41). Hand plate, viewed from the left side. 12 mm CR

1. digital groove	
2. digital ray	
3. dorsum of hand	
4. finger	
5. hand plate	
6. head	
7. nail field	
8. thorax	

212b. Stage 17 (Day 41). 12 mm CR

212c. Stage 18 (Day 44). 16 mm CR

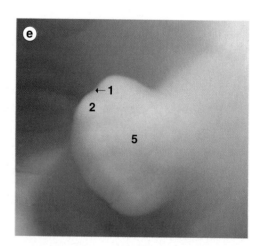

212d. Stage 18 (Day 44). 16 mm CR

212e. Stage 19 (Days 47–48). 18 mm CR

212f. Stage 19 (Days 47–48). Digital rays and grooves are present, view from the left. 20 mm CR

0.5 mm

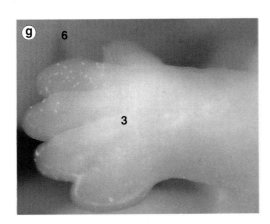

212g. Stage 19 (Days 47–48). Left arm and elbow. The fingers are beginning to separate. 19 mm CR

212i. Stage 22 (Day 54). Fingertips are swollen where the touch pads are developing. 27 mm CR

212h. Stage 22 (Day 54). View from the right. Fingers are separated. 26 mm CR

212j. Week 10. The hands are adducted. Fingernail fields are forming. 60 mm CR ♀

213a. Stage 23 (Days 56–57). Longitudinal section of the index finger. 29 mm CR

1. boundary furrow in epithelium
2. distal phalanx
3. dorsum of finger
4. joint cavity
5. middle phalanx
6. nail bed
7. nail fold

213b–213f. Development of the fingernails.

213b. Week 9. 45 mm CR

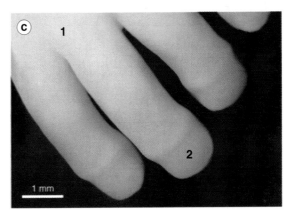

213c. Week 10. 60 mm CR ♀

1. dorsum of hand
2. nail field
3. palm
4. thumb

213d. Week 13. 97 mm CR ♂

1. dorsum of
   hand
2. fingernail
3. nail field
4. thumb

213e. Week 15. 130 mm CR ♀

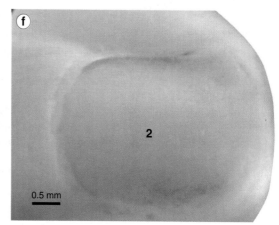

213f. Week 23. Index finger. 220 mm CR ♂

213g–213j. Developing fingers and nails.

213g. Week 8.
34 mm CR

213h. Week 9.
50 mm CR ♀

213i. Week 13.
92 mm CR ♀

213j. Week 15. 123 mm CR ♀

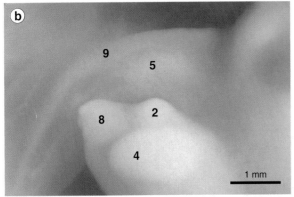

214a–214l.
Development and
rotation of the leg.

214a. Stages 16–17
(Days 37–41).
12 mm CR

1. arm bud
2. genital tubercle
3. head
4. leg bud
5. midgut herniation
6. postaxial border
7. preaxial border
8. tail
9. umbilical cord

LEG DEVELOPMENT AND ROTATION

The lower limb projects 90° from the body (Week 4). The superior surface is called the preaxial border and the inferior surface the postaxial. As the thigh, leg, and foot develop, the foot faces the trunk. The knee then rotates ventrally 90°.

Knee rotation occurs between Weeks 7–9.

At Weeks 10–17 epidermal ridges in the skin form on the plantar surface of the soles and toes.

- The neonatal lower limb tends to remain in its fetal position: the limb is flexed and abducted at the hip joint, the knee flexed, and the foot inverted in the talipes varus position.
- A thick plantar fibrous fat pad conceals the transverse and longitudinal arches of the neonatal sole.
- Congenital dislocation of the hip is not uncommon.
- Only during the second year of postnatal development are the leg and arm equal in length; an increase in leg length is a conspicuous feature of further development.
- Reduction of the limbs (meromelia) or absence of the limbs (amelia) occurs very rarely naturally. Thalidomide can induce these abnormalities.

214b. Higher magnification of **214a**.

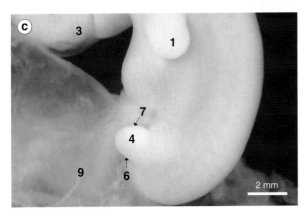

214c. Stages 16–18 (Days 37–44). 14 mm CR

214c and 214d from Dr E.C. Blenkinsopp

214d. Higher magnification of **214c**.

214e. Stages 16–18 (Days 37–44) 14 mm CR

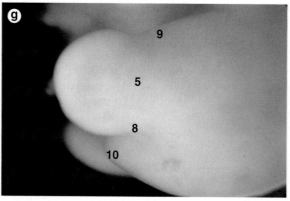

1. foot
2. genital tubercle
3. knee
4. leg
5. leg bud
6. liver
7. midgut herniation
8. postaxial border
9. preaxial border
10. tail
11. thigh
12. toes
13. umbilical cord

214f. Stage 18 (Day 44). 16 mm CR

214g. Stage 19 (Days 47–48). 18 mm CR

214h. Stage 19 (Days 47–48). The knees are forming. 17–20 mm CR

214i. Stage 22 (Day 54). The soles of the feet face each other. 25 mm CR

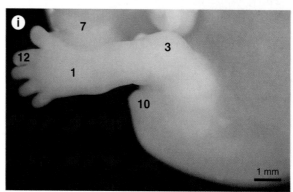

214j. Stage 22 (Day 54). The knee points cranially. 27 mm CR

214k. Stage 22 (Day 54). 27 mm CR

214l. Week 13. 97 mm CR ♂

215a–215d. Early development of the leg and foot.

215a. Stages 14–15 (Days 32–33). Transverse section of the leg bud. 7 mm CR

215a from LHSM

1. apical ectodermal ridge
2. cell death
3. leg bud
4. spinal cord
5. tail
6. toes

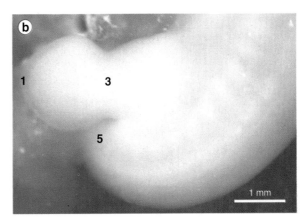

215b. Stages 16–17 (Days 37–41). Note the ectodermal ridge on the leg bud. 12 mm CR

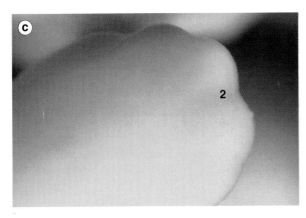

215c. Stage 19 (Days 47–48). Cell death between the developing toes.

215d. Stage 21 (Day 52). The toes are now visible, view of the plantar surface.

216a–216c. Plantar surface (bottom) of the foot.

216a. Stage 22 (Day 54). The great toe bears a similarity in appearance to the thumb. 27 mm CR

1. ankle
2. epidermal ridge
3. plantar surface (sole)
4. toes

216b. Week 9. The great toe has assumed its final position. 50 mm CR ♀

216c. Week 18. Epidermal ridges are present on the sole of the foot. The arches are concealed by a fat pad. 164 mm CR ♂

217a–217c. Development of the toenails.

217a. Week 8. No nail fields are present. 39 mm CR

217b. Week 10. Nail fields are present on the toes. 60 mm CR ♀

217c. Week 24.
228 mm CR ♂

1. ankle
2. dorsum of foot
3. lateral border of foot
4. toenail
5. toenail field

Bones and Joints

BONES

Bone develops either by intracartilaginous (endochondral) or intramembranous ossification.

Endochondral ossification

Initially, the mesoderm forms models of the bones in cartilage. Mesoderm adjacent to the cartilaginous model condenses to form a perichondrium and then periosteum of two layers: an outer fibrous and inner cellular layer. These cartilaginous models grow, principally at the ends, by the chondrocytes in the cartilage increasing in size and also by mitosis.

The long bones of the limbs are examples of intracartilaginous ossification. Ossification begins when chondrocytes in the shaft of the bone mature, phosphatase is produced, and their matrix calcifies. The cavities occupied by late hypertrophic chondrocytes are opened by multinucleate phagocytic cells (chondroclasts), the chondrocytes then die, and their cavities remain.

The inner cellular layer of periosteum then ceases to form chondrocytes, but forms osteoblasts instead. These osteoblasts, along with blood vessels, invade the cavities in the shaft and establish ossification centers. Osteoblasts positioned on the calcified cartilage deposit bone, and ossification spreads up and down the shaft as the chondrocytes die.

The periosteum adds bone to the shaft surface by intramembranous ossification (see below). Bone in the center of the shaft is resorbed and replaced by hemopoietic mesoderm which forms the red marrow. Hemopoiesis begins at about Week 16 in the bone marrow. At Week 10 granulocytes enter the circulation from the bone marrow.

At each extremity of the marrow cavity is a zone of endochondral ossification which advances toward the end of the bone. At the same time, cartilage is deposited at the ends of the bone.

At each end of the bone, one (or more) ossification centers (epiphyses) form. Ossification continues until two types of areas remain: articular cartilage on the extreme ends of the bones and an epiphyseal disc of cartilage between the primary diaphyseal and secondary epiphyseal centers.

Growth of the bone continues at the epiphyseal disc until the mature length is reached and the disc becomes bone.

The epiphyseal plate is divided into four regions (from the diaphyseal plate outward toward the end of the bone): calcified cartilage with degenerating cells (chondrocytes), mature hypertrophic cells in columns, flat proliferating cells, and reserve cells. As the degenerating cells leave their lacunae they are replaced by osteoblasts, which lay bone on the calcified cartilage.

Bones grow in length from the epiphyseal plates and in thickness from the periosteum.

Intramembranous ossification

Mesoderm cells (in flat bones of the skull) differentiate into osteoblasts and form an ossification center. They begin to secrete bone matrix (spicules) and trap the osteoblasts as osteocytes. Osteoblasts surrounding the matrix produce more osteocytes as the bony spicules grow and become more complex. Mesoderm at the periphery of the ossification center forms periosteum. Within the ossification center, osteoclasts appear which resorb or destroy bone.

The growth and ultimate shape of a bone are the result of the combination of deposition of osteoblasts and destruction by osteoclasts. For example, in the frontal bone new bone is added on to the external surface as older bone is destroyed on the internal surface.

- Red marrow is present throughout the neonatal skeleton. After 5 years of age, the red marrow in long bones is gradually replaced by yellow marrow.

218a–218c. Neonatal skull painted to show intramembranous (turquoise) and cartilaginous (dark blue) origins of the bone.

218a. Frontal and lateral view.

218b. Lateral view.

218c. Base of the skull.

1. frontal
2. mandible
3. occipital
4. orbit
5. palatine
6. parietal
7. zygomatic arch

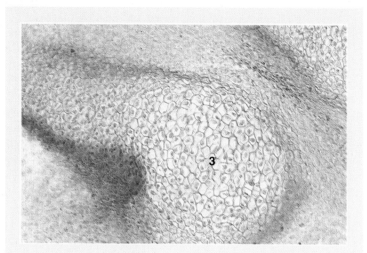

219. Stage 19 (Days 47–48). Developing vertebral spine. 20 mm CR

1. cartilage beginning to hypertrophy in centrum
2. intervertebral disc
3. cartilage beginning to hypertrophy in spine

220a and **220b.** Week 11. Developing vertebrae. **220b** is a higher magnification of **220a**. 29 mm CR

SKELETON

In Weeks 5–6 mesoderm in each limb condenses to form a skeleton which is continuous and has no joints. A cartilaginous center appears in the mesoderm of each bone and the cells differentiate to become cartilage. A cartilaginous model of each bone is formed, while condensed mesoderm surrounding the models forms the perichondrium. The areas between the cartilaginous models are continuous with the perichondrium and will form the joints.

The perichondrium near the center of the shaft of a bone differentiates into a periosteum of two layers. The inner osteogenic layer contains osteoblasts, which lay down bone matrix and fibers on the shaft. Calcium salts from the blood are then deposited and bone tissue is formed as a cylinder around the cartilaginous model.

221a–221d.
Developing skeleton in the hand.

221a. Stage 19 (Days 47–48) 20 mm CR

221b. Week 13. 95 mm CR

1. dorsum of hand
2. cartilaginous bone primordium
3. joint
4. mesodermal metacarpal primordia
5. metacarpals
6. palm of hand
7. skin
8. thumb

221c. Week 8. Developing finger bone. 40 mm CR

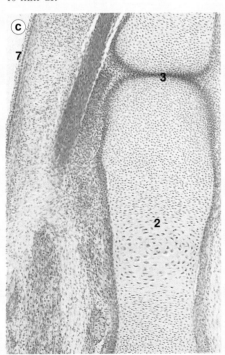

221d. Week 11. Developing skeleton of the forearm and hand. 65 mm CR

222a–222c. Developing skeleton in the leg.

222a. Stage 19 (Days 47–48). 20 mm CR

222b. Week 8. 35 mm CR

222c. Week 9. 48 mm CR ♀

1. genital tubercle
2. greater saphenous vein
3. knee
4. leg bud
5. mesodermal metatarsal primordia
6. tibia

JOINTS

Joints form in Weeks 6–8.

Synovial joints

Mesoderm surrounding the joint area condenses to form a capsule which is continuous with the shaft perichondrium and ligaments. Each bone end in the joint is covered by a layer of dense mesoderm, which will form the articular cartilages and synovial membranes. Within the joint capsule, fluid spaces appear in the loose mesoderm. These join to form the joint cavity.

Fibrocartilaginous joints

The mesoderm in the joint differentiates to form fibrocartilage (e.g., the symphysis pubis) or hyaline cartilage (e.g., the neurocentral joint).

Fibrous joints

The mesoderm in the joint differentiates to form dense fibrous connective tissue (e.g., the frontal or metopic suture of the skull).

223. Left knee of a full-term fetus dissected and viewed from the front. The femur has been removed and the patella is reflected forward.

1. femur
2. fibula
3. patella
4. synovial folds
5. tibia

223 from RCS

224a and **224b.** Early sternum. View of the ventral surface.

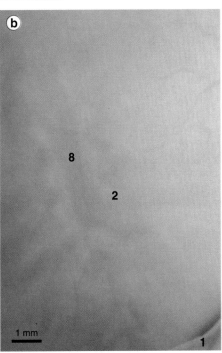

224a. Stage 22 (Day 54). The two sternal bars. 27 mm CR

224b. Week 10. 57 mm CR ♂

Sternum

Mesodermal condensations form two widely separated sternal bars in the thorax. During Week 9 the two sternal bars, which are approximately parallel in the midline, fuse to one another cephalo-caudally to form cartilaginous models of the manubrium, body, and xiphoid process. These bars are connected to the ends of the costal cartilages.

Centers of ossification appear cephalo-caudally during Weeks 20–25, except in the xiphoid process.

- In the neonate, the manubrium usually contains one main center of ossification, the upper segments of the body usually contain one main center, and the lower segments contain paired centers. Ossification of the lowest segments begins shortly after birth and that of the xiphoid process during the third year of life.
- If fusion is incomplete a minor fissure or perforation may be present in the sternum.

---

1. arm
2. costal cartilages
3. face
4. hand
5. liver bulge
6. rib
7. sternal bars
8. sternum
9. umbilical cord

225a and **225b.** Centers of ossification in the sternum.

225a. Weeks 20–24. Four centers of ossification are present: one in the manubrium (removed) and three in the body.

225b. Weeks 20–24. The specimen has been injected, dried, and preserved in oil.

1. body of sternum
2. internal thoracic artery
3. manubrium sterni
4. ossification centers
5. rib
6. xiphoid process

225a and 225b from RCS

Ribs

The mesoderm models of the ribs form from the costal processes of the thoracic vertebrae. They become cartilaginous, and during Weeks 13–14 a primary ossification center appears in the body of the rib.

- In the neonate, the ribs are more horizontal and less curved than those in the adult.
- Breathing in the neonate is primarily due to the musculature of the diaphragm and the abdominal wall.
- At puberty secondary centers of ossification appear for the head and tubercle of the rib.

1. arm bud and hand plate (paddle)
2. cactus needle and reflected skin
3. ear
4. elbow
5. eye
6. forebrain
7. hand
8. heart bulge
9. hindbrain
10. leg
11. leg bud
12. liver bulge
13. midgut herniation
14. precartilaginous rib
15. rib
16. umbilical cord

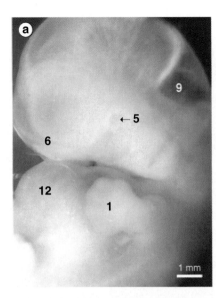

226a–226e. Developing ribs.

226a. Stage 17 (Day 41). Ribs are not present on the ventral surface at this stage. 12 mm CR

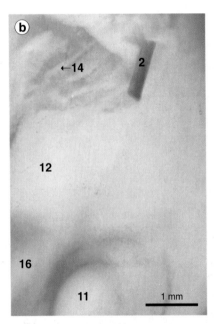

226b. Stages 17–18 (Days 41–44). Precartilaginous ribs are present. 14 mm CR

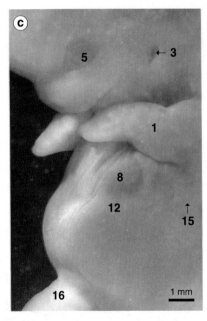

226c. Stage 19 (Days 47–48). The ribs have grown partly around the body wall. 20 mm CR

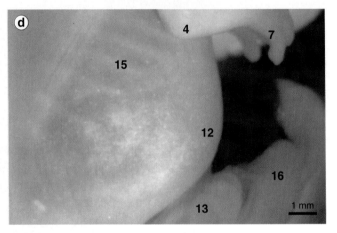

226d. Stage 22 (Day 54). 27 mm CR

226e. Stage 23 (Days 56–57). 27 mm CR

227. Week 8. Inner aspect of the ribs and costal cartilages. 40 mm CR ♀

1. costal cartilages
2. rib
3. ventricle of heart

Pelvis

The neonatal pelvis is more vertical than that in the adult and does not exhibit any sexual differences.

At birth the majority of the body of the ilium, the ramus of the ischium, and the superior ramus of the pubis are ossified. They are separated by a 'Y' shaped cartilage forming the bulk of the acetabulum. The head of the femur is normally larger than the acetabulum and extends beyond its margins.

● When the infant walks (second year), the sacrum descends between the ilia.

228. Full-term pelvis. Note the radiating ossific fibers in the ilium. The coccyx is still completely cartilaginous. ♀

1. coccyx
2. ilium
3. iliac crest
4. ischium
5. pubis
6. 'Y' shaped epiphyseal plate

228 from RCS

5 mm

Skull and arch derivatives

The skull consists of the neurocranium, which protects the brain, and the skeleton of the jaws (viscerocranium). The basal part of the skull is cartilaginous, i.e., the occipital bone, body of the sphenoid, lesser wings of the sphenoid, body of the ethmoid, otic capsules, nasal capsules, and the petrous and mastoid parts of the temporals.

The flat bones of the skull are membranous, i.e., the frontals and parietals, the squamous parts of the temporals and occipitals, and the nasal and the lacrimal bones.

The skeleton of the jaws (or viscerocranium) is also formed by cartilaginous and membranous ossification. The cartilaginous parts form from the first and second branchial arches by mesoderm condensing to form a rod of cartilage. Some of the cartilage or its perichondrium is retained to form adult structures, but most is later replaced by membranous bone.

The membranous parts of the viscerocranium include the maxillary prominence of the first branchial arch, which forms the maxilla, the zygomatic and squamous parts of the temporal, the vomer, and the palatine bone. The mandible forms around the ventral end of the first arch cartilage (Meckel's cartilage). Some cartilaginous ossification occurs at the mandibular condyle and the center of the chin.

As the brain grows the flat bones of the skull grow to accommodate it by the deposition of new bone on the external surface and by the destruction of old bone on the internal surface.

In arches three to six, cartilage bars only form at the ventral end of the arch. Cartilage at the dorsal end of arch one (Meckel's cartilage) forms the malleus and incus; cartilage at the dorsal end of arch two (Reichert's cartilage) forms the stapes and styloid process; and cartilage at the ventral end of arch two forms the lesser cornu and upper body of the hyoid bone. Arch three cartilage (ventral end) forms the greater cornu and lower body of the hyoid. Arches four and six fuse to form the laryngeal cartilages, with the exception of the epiglottis (formed from the hypobranchial eminence of arches three and four).

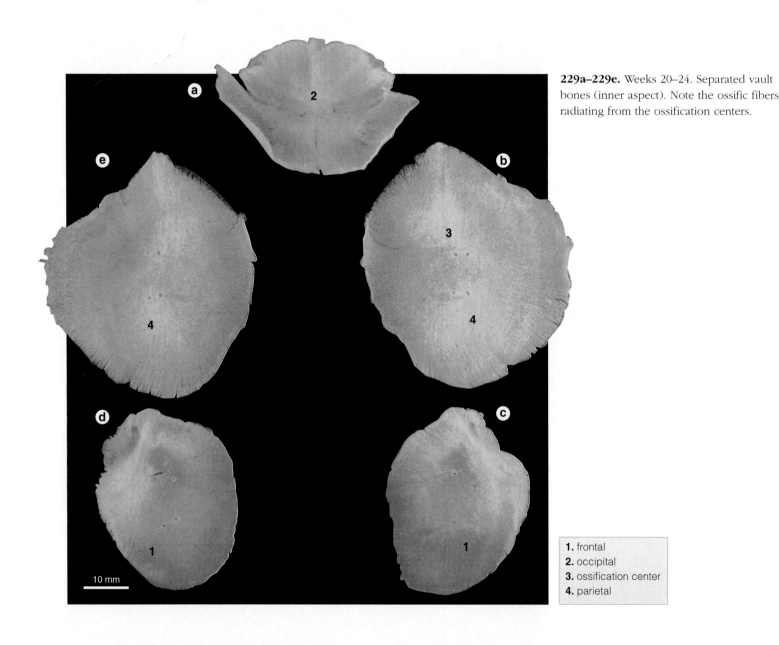

229a–229e. Weeks 20–24. Separated vault bones (inner aspect). Note the ossific fibers radiating from the ossification centers.

10 mm

1. frontal
2. occipital
3. ossification center
4. parietal

NEONATAL SKULL

The neonatal face is approximately one-eighth of the total cranium. This ratio changes in the adult to approximately one-half. The small face in the neonate is due to the lack of erupted teeth, and to the small size of the nasal cavity and maxillary sinuses.

The flat bones of the skull are separated by fibrous membranes called sutures. Expansions in the sutures are called fontanelles. There are normally six fontanelles present at birth. The diamond-shaped anterior fontanelle is approximately 25 mm in diameter, and the skin overlying it pulsates. This fontanelle is obliterated by the progressive ingrowing of the borders of the membranous bone. This process begins about 3 months after birth, and the fontanelle is usually obliterated by the second year. The posterior, two sphenoidal, and two mastoidal fontanelles are obliterated between 6 months and 2 years after birth. Numerous accessory fontanelles may also be present. Palpation of the fontanelles allows clinical evaluation of hydration, intracranial pressure and bone growth.

Most of the bones of the skull are ossified at birth, but move relative to one another at the sutures because the bones are soft and loosely connected. This mobility is particularly important in childbirth since it allows the bones to overlap. The parietals overlap the frontals, though the frontals do not overlap each other, as they are fixed at the root of the nose. The parietals also overlap the occipitals, and one parietal is driven under the other (see Childbirth).

The mastoid process does not develop until the second year, and the facial nerve is relatively exposed and unprotected as it emerges from the stylomastoid foramen. In a difficult delivery, forceps may damage the nerve.

- The neonate lacks superciliary arches.
- The skull continues to grow rapidly in the first 2 years after birth. New bone is added at the edges of the bones.

Mandible

The neonatal mandible is composed of two halves united by a midline suture (symphysis menti). The two halves fuse by the beginning of the second year.

The angle of the rami is broad (140°) and the mandibular notch is shallow.

Ten large alveolar fossae, each containing a deciduous tooth, are present.

- In the young adult, the angle of the ramus is 120° or less, while in the elderly the angle becomes broader again due to resorption of bone.
- Diploë form around the age of 2 years.

Maxilla

The neonatal maxilla is low in height and its increase vertically in the child is due to an increase in size of the maxillary sinus and alveolar portion.

At birth, the infraorbital foramina are large and the alveolar portion contains ten large alveoli with deciduous teeth.

Occipital bone

The occipital bone at birth is composed of four parts separated by cartilage: a squamous part, two lateral parts, and a basilar part. All the parts are usually fused by the fourth year.

Sphenoid

The neonatal sphenoid is composed of three parts: a single middle portion and two lateral parts each consisting of part of the greater wing and the medial pterygoid plate which unite during the first year. The sphenoidal sinuses invade the sphenoid at 5 years of age.

Temporal bone

The newborn temporal bones are in three parts: squamous, petrous, and tympanic. The mastoid process is absent and the styloid process is largely cartilaginous.

The tympanic part of the bone is an incomplete bony ring.

- The petrosquamous fissure separating the petrous and squamous temporal bone is a potential pathway for infection into the mastoid antrum of the middle ear.

Frontal bone

The two frontal bones fuse by 6–8 years and their suture is rarely present in the adult. The frontal sinuses are absent at birth and invade the bones at about 2 years of age.

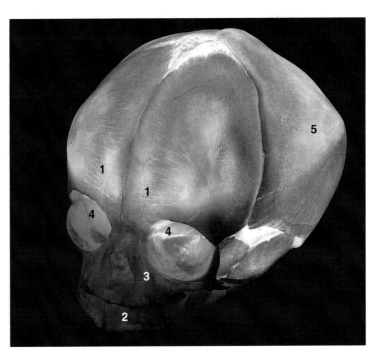

230. The neonatal skull illuminated by transmitted light. Note the thinness of the bones of the vault.

1. frontal
2. mandible
3. maxilla
4. orbit
5. parietal

231a–231c. Neonatal skull.

231a. View of the left side.

231b. View of the left front.

231c. View of the back.

10 mm

1. anterior fontanelle
2. coronal suture
3. deciduous teeth elevation
4. external acoustic meatus
5. frontal bone
6. frontal suture
7. frontal tuberosity
8. lambdoid suture
9. mandible
10. mastoid fontanelle
11. maxilla
12. occipital bone
13. orbit
14. parietal bone
15. parietal tuberosity
16. posterior fontanelle
17. sagittal suture
18. sphenoidal fontanelle
19. stylomastoid foramen
20. symphysis menti
21. tympanic ring
22. zygomatic arch

Vertebral column

During Week 4 sclerotome cells from the somites surround the (1) ventromedial aspect of the notochord, to form the centrum and intervertebral disc, (2) dorsal to the neural tube, and (3) ventrolateral aspect of the body wall, to form the costal processes. In the thorax these form ribs. Those cells ventromedial to the notochord arrange themselves in alternating bands of loose and densely packed cells. The centrum of a vertebra is formed when a region of packed cells fuses with a region of loose cells immediately caudal which has arisen from an adjacent sclerotome. Some densely packed cells from each region also migrate cranially opposite the myotome to form the intervertebral disc. The intersegmental nerves lie close to the discs, while the arteries lie close to the bodies.

The notochord persists as the nucleus pulposus of the intervertebral disc but disappears in the vertebral body.

Chondrification begins in Week 6. Ossification begins before birth and ends during the 25th year. At birth three primary centers are present: in the centrum and in each half of the vertebral arch.

- During years 3–5 the two halves of the vertebral arch fuse.
- Joints between the arch and centrum allow the spinal cord to enlarge. When the arch fuses with the centrum between 3–6 years of age, these joints disappear.
- The thoracic vertebral column gradually develops a relatively fixed curve after birth.
- The cervical curve appears when the infant begins to lift its head.
- The lumbar curve appears at the end of the first year, when the infant begins to walk.

232. Week 19. Sagittal section of the vertebral column *in situ.*

1. arm
2. cerebellum
3. cerebral hemisphere
4. heart
5. intestine
6. leg
7. liver
8. nasal cavity
9. tongue
10. umbilical cord
11. vertebral column

233. Dissected neonatal vertebral column.

1. cervical vertebrae
2. lumbar vertebrae
3. sacral vertebrae
4. thoracic vertebrae

10 mm

10 mm

232 from RCS

233 from RFHSM

Developmental series (alizarin red stain)

The cartilaginous or membranous skeleton is ossified when discrete centers of ossification appear. The first center occurs in the clavicle and then in the jaws and palate at Week 7, and in the frontal bone at Weeks 8–9.

The skeletons of embryos and fetuses can be stained with alizarin red and the other body tissues cleared. Such preparations show the ossification centers and demonstrate the progress of ossification in the body.

- In the female, the centers of ossification appear before those in the male and complete their ossification first.
- At birth all bones in the skeleton have red marrow (centers of hemopoiesis). In the adult hemopoiesis is limited to the red marrow of cancellous bone, i.e., the ribs, sternum, vertebral bodies, femur, humerus, and diploë of the skull.
- The calcanial center of ossification (Weeks 16–20) is used medico-legally to establish maturity.

234a–234r. Primary ossification centers demonstrated by alizarin red staining and clearing.

234a. Stages 17–18 (Days 41–44).

1. clavicle
2. femur
3. fibula
4. frontal
5. humerus
6. ilium
7. mandible
8. maxilla
9. parietal
10. radius
11. ribs
12. scapula
13. tibia
14. ulna

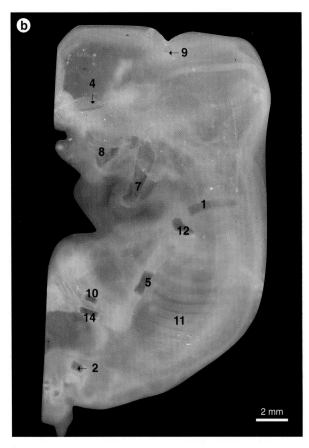

234b. Stage 22 (Day 54).

234c. Week 8.

234a–234c from RCS

234d. Week 11. The specimen has been stretched during mounting.

234d and *234f* from RFHSM

234e. Week 11.

234e from RCS

234f. Weeks 11–12.

234g. Week 13.

234g and 234i from RFHSM

234h. Weeks 13–14. This specimen has been damaged during preparation.

234h from RCS

234i. Week 13.

1. clavicle
2. femur
3. fibula
4. frontal
5. humerus
6. ilium
7. mandible
8. maxilla
9. occipital
10. parietal
11. radius
12. ribs
13. scapula
14. tibia
15. ulna

234j. Week 14. This specimen has been stretched in preparation.

234j from RFHSM

234k. Week 14.

234k from RCS

234l. Week 15.

234l from Dr D. Dooley

1. femur	
2. fibula	
3. frontal	
4. humerus	
5. ilium	
6. mandible	
7. maxilla	
8. parietal	
9. phalanges	
10. radius	
11. ribs	
12. scapula	
13. tibia	
14. ulna	

ⓜ

10 mm

234m. Week 16.

234m–234o from RCS

ⓝ

10 mm

234n. Week 16.

ⓞ

10 mm

234o. Week 17.

| 1. calcaneum |
| 2. clavicle |
| 3. femur |
| 4. fibula |
| 5. frontal |
| 6. humerus |
| 7. ilium |
| 8. mandible |
| 9. maxilla |
| 10. parietal |
| 11. radius |
| 12. ribs |
| 13. scapula |
| 14. tibia |
| 15. ulna |

(p)

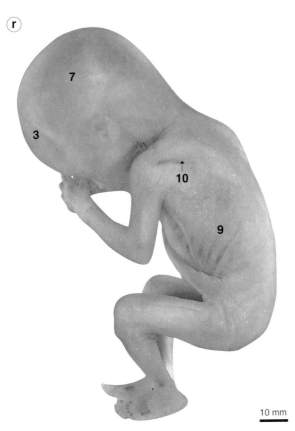

(r)

234p. Week 18.

234p from RCS

234q. Week 18.

234q and 234r from RFHSM

234r. Same specimen as in **234q**. After Week 18 the ossification centers become obscured by the muscles.

1. femur
2. fibula
3. frontal
4. humerus
5. mandible
6. maxilla
7. parietal
8. radius
9. ribs
10. scapula
11. tibia
12. ulna

Fetal skeleton

235. A fetus *in utero.*

1. femur
2. fibula
3. frontal
4. humerus
5. mandible
6. maxilla
7. parietal
8. radius
9. ribs
10. tibia
11. ulna
12. vertebrae

235 from Mr J. Bashford, J.D. Boyd Collection

236. A disarticulated full-term skeleton.

1. calcaneum
2. carpals
3. centrum
4. cervical vertebrae
5. clavicle
6. coccyx
7. conchae
8. deciduous teeth
9. ear ossicles and tympanic ring
10. femur
11. fibula
12. frontal
13. humerus
14. ilium
15. ischium
16. lumbar vertebrae
17. mandible
18. maxilla
19. metacarpals
20. proximal phalanx
21. nasal
22. occipital
23. palatine
24. parietal
25. petrous temporal
26. distal phalanx
27. pubis
28. radius
29. ribs
30. sacral vertebrae
31. scapula
32. sphenoid
33. talus
34. metatarsals
35. thoracic vertebrae
36. tibia
37. ulna
38. vomer
39. zygomatic bone
40. zygomatic process and squamous temporal

236 from RFHSM

237a. Weeks 13–16.

237b. Weeks 17–24. Fetal ribs are almost horizontal.

237c. Weeks 21–28.

237a–237e. Articulated fetal skeleton to demonstrate relative size differences. The legs have been extended and adducted.

1. cervical vertebrae
2. femur
3. fibula
4. foot
5. hand
6. humerus
7. lumbar vertebrae
8. pelvis
9. ribs
10. skull
11. tibia

237d. Weeks 25–32. The fetal skull is as wide as the pectoral girdle.

237e. Weeks 29–36.

237a–237e from RFHSM

238. Full-term fetal skeleton in the normal position *in utero.*

1. ear
2. femur
3. foot
4. frontal
5. hand
6. humerus
7. ilium
8. parietal
9. radius
10. ribs
11. scapula
12. ulna
13. vertebral column

10 mm

238 from RFHSM

Fetal radiology

239a. Week 9. Anteroposterior radiograph of a male fetus with a foot length of 6 mm.

239b. Week 12. Lateral radiograph of a male fetus with a foot length of 15 mm.

239c. Week 29. Anteroposterior radiograph of a female fetus with a foot length of 60 mm.

239a–239c from Mr J. Bashford, J.D. Boyd Collection

1. acromion
2. anterior fontanelle
3. clavicle
4. external auditory meatus
5. frontal
6. humerus
7. mandible
8. parietal
9. rib
10. femur
11. ileum
12. metacarpals
13. metatarsals
14. proximal phalanges
15. pubis
16. radius
17. ulna
18. vertebrae

Muscles

Muscles form from myoblasts which have differentiated from mesoderm, except for those of the iris which are derived from ectoderm.

Skeletal muscles form primarily from the myotome region of somites, but some head and neck muscles are formed from branchial arch myoblasts. Somatic mesoderm forms limb muscles *in situ*.

Each myotome divides into dorsal and ventral parts and as the spinal nerve develops it sends a branch to each part: the dorsal and ventral primary rami. The myoblasts then migrate to their final positions although some muscles remain segmentally arranged, e.g., the intercostals.

Most smooth muscles and cardiac muscles form from splanchnic mesoderm. The first heartbeats occur during Weeks 3–4.

At Week 7 some of the neck and trunk muscles begin to contract spontaneously, arm and leg movements then occur and are detectable by ultrasound methods. By Week 12 the fetus can respond to skin stimulation and some postural reflexes are also present.

By Weeks 16–20 the fetal movements are felt by the mother, a phenomenon known as 'quickening'.

240a.
Stage 10.
Transverse section of a 10 somite embryo.

1. amnion
2. amniotic cavity
3. neural tube
4. somite

240a from J.D. Boyd Collection

240b. Stage 17 (Day 41). The muscles are represented by the somites. The thoracic, abdominal, and tail region of a 12 mm CR embryo.

1. arm
2. arm bud
3. ear
4. eye
5. head
6. leg bud
7. liver bulge
8. somites
9. superficial temporal artery
10. tail
11. umbilical cord

5 mm

241. Week 13. In addition to swallowing amniotic fluid, a fetus may suck a finger from approximately Week 11. 92 mm CR ♀

SWALLOWING REFLEXES

At Week 11 the fetus will open its mouth if the oral region is stimulated and suck a finger. At Week 12 the fetus regularly swallows amniotic fluid, and near term it is swallowing approximately 750 ml daily. In addition to the fluid, numerous other materials are swallowed, e.g., sloughed cells from the skin, oral cavity and respiratory tract, lanugo hairs, and *vernix caseosa*.

Integument

EPIDERMIS

The epidermis forms from ectoderm and the dermis forms from mesoderm associated with the ectoderm.

The epidermis is a simple epithelium at Week 4, but by Week 7 a superficial layer of periderm is present, which keratinizes and desquamates. Cells are replaced by the basal layer, the stratum germinativum. At Week 11 an intermediate layer forms from cells of the stratum germinativum. All of the adult layers are present at birth. Until approximately Week 17 the skin is very thin and the underlying blood vessels are visible.

The desquamated periderm cells together with sebum from sebaceous glands, lanugo hairs, and amniotic cells form a white protective covering (*vernix caseosa*) for the fetal skin. This is primarily found on the back, on hair, and in joint creases. It also fills the external auditory meatus at birth. From Week 21 the periderm cells gradually disappear and desquamated epidermal cells replace them in the *vernix caseosa*.

During Weeks 13–17 downgrowths of stratum germinativum penetrate into the dermis, producing epidermal ridges which appear on the palmar surfaces of the hands and fingers and the plantar surfaces of the feet and toes. Each individual has a distinctive pattern.

- Epidermal ridge patterns can be used diagnostically to indicate abnormal chromosome complements.

MELANOCYTES

Around Week 8, melanoblasts migrate from the neural crest to the basal layer of the epidermis and form melanocytes. Melanin is produced before birth.

242a–242c. Development of the skin, samples taken from the arm above the elbow.

242a. Week 10. 60 mm CR ♀ **242b.** Week 13. 101 mm CR ♀ **242c.** Week 23. 220 mm CR ♂

1. developing collagenous and elastic fibers (dermis)	**3.** intermediate layer	**5.** stratum corneum	**7.** stratum lucidum
2. epidermal ridge	**4.** periderm	**6.** stratum granulosum	**8.** stratum spinosum and germinativum

243. Week 13. The skin is very thin and the developing blood vessels are easily distinguished. Note the lack of *vernix caseosa*. 97 mm CR ♂

1. arm
2. back
3. eye
4. hand
5. superficial temporal artery

10 mm

DERMIS

The dermis originates from somatic mesoderm and the dermomyotome part of the somites. At Week 11, elastic and collagenous fibers are produced.

- Down's syndrome can be recognized by an abnormal epidermal ridge pattern, e.g., there is only one palmar crease rather than the normal two.
- Neonates of dark-skinned races are only slightly darker than those of white-skinned races. After birth, their skin darkens due to increased melanin production in response to light. In the sacral region, pigmented dermal melanocytes appear as a slate-blue or 'Mongolian' spot, which disappears during the first year of life.

244a and **244b.** *Vernix caseosa* on the face and scalp.

244a. Week 18. 152 mm CR ♂

244b. Week 18. *Vernix caseosa* on the back of the head. 160 mm CR ♀

1. ear
2. eye
3. eyebrow
4. lanugo
5. nose
6. scalp
7. *vernix caseosa*

245a and **245b.** Week 13. Dermal ridges on the thumb.

1. dermal ridges
2. distal phalanx of thumb
3. fingernail
4. palmar surface

245a. 101 mm CR ♀

245b. Higher magnification of the palmar surface of the thumb in **245a.**

HAIR

Hair follicles form (Weeks 9–12) when downgrowths from the stratum germinativum penetrate into the dermis. The ends form hair bulbs containing the germinal matrices which produce the hairs. Melanocytes differentiate in the bulb from melanoblasts. Melanin is transferred from the melanocytes to the germinal matrix before birth. A hair papilla (mesoderm) invaginates the base of each hair bulb. The root sheath forms: the epithelial part from the hair follicle and the dermal portion from surrounding mesoderm.

The germinal matrix proliferates and the hair shaft cells are pushed up, keratinize, pierce the epidermis, and protrude above the skin surface. Arrector pili muscles form from surrounding mesoderm.

Very fine hairs or lanugo first appear on the eyebrows, chin, and upper lip, followed by the forehead and scalp, and by Week 20 cover most of the body. Lanugo is replaced by secondary hairs (vellus), arising from new hair follicles. By Weeks 26–29, the secondary hair on the head is longer than the lanugo, which is being shed. The new hair follicles cover almost all of the body.

- Lanugo is from the Latin *lana*, meaning fine wool.
- Lanugo is shed before and shortly after birth, the last parts being shed from the eyelashes, eyebrows, and scalp.

SEBACEOUS GLANDS

Most of the sebaceous glands form as buds from a hair follicle root sheath, except for those of the glans penis and the labia minora, which bud from the epidermis. The sebaceous gland buds form several alveoli and ducts. The central alveolar cells break down to form oily sebum, which is released into the hair follicle, onto the skin, and so forms part of the *vernix caseosa*.

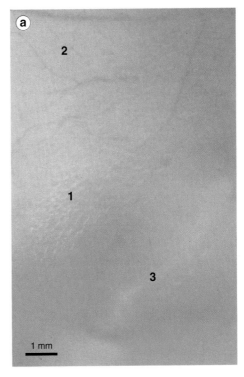

246a and **246b.** Development of the eyebrow viewed from the front.

1. eyebrow
2. forehead
3. fused eyelid
4. lanugo

1 mm

246a. Week 13. 97 mm CR ♂

246b. Week 15. 130 mm CR ♀

2 mm

247. Week 13. Transverse paraffin wax section of the eyebrow. 101 mm CR ♀

1. blood vessels in hair papilla
2. bulb
3. dermal root sheath
4. hair shaft

248. Week 17. Lanugo hairs on the face. 150 mm CR ♀

1. eye
2. forehead
3. lanugo

249a and **249b.** Lanugo and vellus hairs.

249a. Week 20. Scalp showing both lanugo and scalp hairs, view from the right side. 185 mm CR ♀

1. hair
2. head
3. lanugo

249b. Week 22. Scalp covered with scalp hairs and *vernix caseosa*, view from behind. 210 mm CR ♂

1. crown of head
2. hair
3. *vernix caseosa*

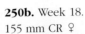

250a and **250b.**
Developing
mammary gland
in transverse
paraffin wax
sections.

250a. Week 18.
152 mm CR ♂

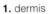

250b. Week 18.
155 mm CR ♀

1. dermis
2. developing
   mammary
   gland
3. mammary pit
4. secondary
   bud

SWEAT GLANDS

Merocrine sweat glands form (Week 20) as solid epidermal downgrowths into the dermis, the tip becoming a coiled gland and the stalk a duct. The lumen of the sweat gland forms by canalization; the peripheral cells form secretory and myoepithelial cells (smooth muscle).

Apocrine sweat glands bud from the epithelial downgrowths which will form the hair follicles.

TEETH

For Teeth, see Lips and teeth.

FINGERNAILS AND TOENAILS

For fingernails and toenails, see Limbs.

MAMMARY GLAND

At the beginning of Week 4 a ridge of thickened ectoderm extends from the axilla to the inguinal region. During Week 6 it thickens and becomes depressed in the pectoral region. Numerous secondary epithelial lactiferous cords (Week 13) then grow from it into the underlying mesoderm, and at Weeks 32–36 the downgrowths and the cords become canalized. The nipples are depressed and poorly formed by birth.

- Either at full-term or in the neonatal period, the nipple is formed when a proliferation of mesoderm beneath the downgrowth elevates it above the adjacent skin.
- At birth, the mammary glands have the same appearance in either sex.
- As a result of maternal sex hormones crossing the placenta, the breast in either sex may, for the first few days following birth, secrete a milky substance known as 'witches milk'.
- As the thorax grows in childhood, the two nipples move further away from the midline.
- In the female at puberty, estrogen stimulates further duct growth and the deposition of fat.

251a–251d.
Developing
nipple.

251a. Stage 22
(Day 54).
27 mm CR

251b. Week 9.
48 mm CR ♀

1. arm
2. eye
3. hand
4. head
5. nipple (areola)
6. nose
7. thorax

251c. Week 13.
97 mm CR ♂

251d. Week 18.
164 mm CR ♂

Fat Deposition

Around Week 27 subcutaneous fat storage commences and the body becomes plump. Two colors of fat may be distinguished: white (yellow) and brown. Brown adipose tissue forms in Weeks 17–20 and is important in metabolism and heat production. It is present at the root of the neck, in the perirenal area, behind the sternum, around the organs in the thorax, and on the posterior abdominal wall.

- A fetus born prematurely at Weeks 25–26 looks old and wizened due to the lack of subcutaneous fat and the fact that the skin grows faster than the underlying connective tissue.
- Fat also accumulates in the cheeks, forming 'buccal fat pads' over the buccinator muscles which prevent the cheeks being drawn in during suckling.
- At birth, the neonatal temperature is the same or slightly higher than the mother's, but it then immediately drops below hers.

252a–252c. The deposition of white (yellow) fat.

1. buccal fat pad
2. chin
3. ear
4. eye
5. fat
6. mouth
7. neck
8. nose
9. parotid gland
10. platysma muscle (cut)
11. shoulder

252a. Week 18. Buccal fat pad. 152 mm CR ♂

252b and **252c.** Distribution of white (yellow) fat on the neck, shoulders, and back.

252b. Week 17. 110 mm CR

252c. Week 18. 152 mm CR ♂

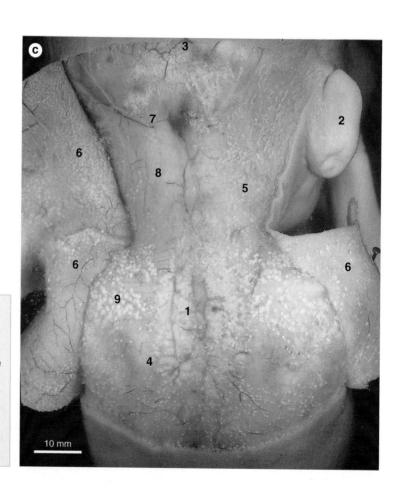

1. fat deposited in a pad
2. ear
3. head
4. medial border of the scapula
5. neck
6. reflected skin
7. superior nuchal line
8. trapezius muscle
9. white fat

Lymphatics

The lymphatic system develops at the end of Week 5. Two pairs of lymph sacs develop, the jugular sacs and the iliac sacs. Two single sacs also form: the retroperitoneal sac and the cisterna chyli. Lymphatic vessels grow out from these sacs and spread throughout the body. They join one another to form a network and also connect to the venous system. During the early fetal period, the lymph sacs (except part of the cisterna chyli) are converted into lymph nodes.

THE LUNG

Mesoderm surrounding the sacs invades them and forms the connective tissue framework and capsule of the lymph nodes. Lymphocytes invade from the thymus. Later, some lymphocytes form from the node mesoderm.

- Lymphoid nodules and germinal centers appear shortly after birth.
- During the first hours after birth lymph flow in the lungs is fast.

TONSILS

The lingual tonsils form from lymph nodules in the root of the tongue, the palatine tonsils from the second pharyngeal pouch, the tubal tonsils from lymph nodules around the auditory (Eustachian) tubes, and the pharyngeal tonsils (adenoids) from lymph nodules in the nasopharynx.

- The pharyngeal tonsil reaches its maximum size at the age of 6 years and usually involutes by puberty.
- The palatine tonsil atrophies between 5 years and puberty.

SPLEEN

For the Spleen, see p. 126.

253a and **235b.** The developing lymph nodes.

0.5 mm

253a. Week 9. Developing axillary lymph node, view of the ventral surface. 50 mm CR ♀

1. arm
2. lymph node
3. thorax

253b. Stage 22 (Day 54). A developing lymph node in the neck. 25 mm CR

1. bronchus
2. lymph node

Growth of the Pregnant Uterus

The non-pregnant uterus lies within the pelvis.

During pregnancy, the uterus expands due to hypertrophy of the existing muscle fibers and the addition of some new ones. In the first trimester the uterus reaches the level of the umbilicus and by Weeks 28–30 it is in the epigastric region.

254. Full-term fetus
in utero.

10 mm

254 *from RCS*

1. abdomen
2. arm
3. cervix (maternal)
4. head
5. leg
6. ovary (maternal)
7. uterus (maternal)

Childbirth

255a *from CCHMS*

255a. Second stage of labor, with the cervix dilated and the occiput of the head below the symphysis pubis.

There are three stages of labor, the first of which extends from the onset of labor until there is complete dilatation of the cervix. At the start of the first stage a blood-stained mucous discharge occurs, then the amnion and chorion form a wedge known as the 'bag of waters' which dilates the internal os. As the internal os dilates, the cervix is shortened or 'taken up' into the lower uterine segment. Late in the first stage, the wedge of amnion and chorion ruptures and the amniotic fluid lying in front of the advancing head escapes as the 'forewaters'. Regular contractions are then established less than 10 minutes apart and the cervix dilates completely. The first stage lasts about 10–12 h in primigravidae or about 7 h or less in multigravidae.

The second stage of labor begins when the cervix is completely dilated and ends with the delivery of the fetus. This stage lasts about 30–90 minutes in primigravidae and 20 minutes or less in multigravidae. As the amniotic fluid has escaped, the uterine contractions can act directly on the fetus forcing it down the birth canal and through the vagina. If the head presents in a vertex presentation, it undergoes the following movements: engagement when the head passes the pelvic brim, descent, flexion of the head on the body pressing the chin against the chest, internal rotation, a spiral movement which starts when the head reaches the pelvic floor and continues during its descent until complete rotation occurs with the occiput usually rotating forward; extension of the head occurs as it escapes from the birth canal, flexion of the head occurs after the face and chin pass the perineum, and, finally, as the head is born the trunk descends into the pelvis, the shoulders are rotated into the anteroposterior diameter of the outlet, and the birth of the trunk and legs follows quickly. The remaining liquor amnii then escapes.

The third stage of labor, which lasts 5–25 minutes begins with the birth of the baby and ends with the delivery of the placenta and membranes. As the uterus continues to contract and to retract, the placenta separates from the uterine wall, more of the umbilical cord appears, and the placenta and membranes are delivered. During the recovery stage, sometimes referred to as the fourth stage of labor, the spiral arteries constrict with further myometrial contractions.

1. abdomen
2. arm
3. back
4. buttock
5. cervix (maternal)
6. head
7. leg
8. placenta
9. umbilical cord
10. uterus (maternal)

255b *from CCHMS*

1. cervix
2. placenta
3. uterus

255b. Third stage of labor, with the placenta beginning to separate from the uterine wall.

256a–256f. Descent and delivery of the fetal skull in the bony birth canal.

256a. The head is presenting in the transverse diameter of the pelvic brim.

256b and **256c.** Descent, engagement, and internal rotation of the head.

1. acetabulum
2. anterior superior iliac spine
3. body of pubis
4. external acoustic meatus (fetal)
5. foramen magnum (fetal)
6. frontal (fetal)
7. hard palate (fetal)
8. iliac fossa
9. ischial tuberosity
10. ischiopubic ramus
11. mandible (fetal)
12. occipital (fetal)
13. orbit (fetal)
14. parietal (fetal)
15. sacrum

20 mm

256d. Delivery and extension of the head.

ⓓ

256e. The head rotates to a natural position relative to its shoulders (restitution).

256f. External rotation of the head.

1. acetabulum
2. anterior fontanelle (fetal)
3. anterior superior iliac spine
4. body of pubis
5. frontal (fetal)
6. iliac fossa
7. ischial tuberosity
8. occipital (fetal)
9. parietal (fetal)
10. sacrum

20 mm

Glossary

Abduction Movement away from the midline of the body.

Abortion Pregnancy ending before viability (20 weeks). Spontaneous (naturally occurring) abortions usually occur in the first 12 weeks. Therapeutic abortions are those induced purposefully.

Adduction Movement toward the midline of the body.

Afterbirth At birth the umbilical cord, placenta, amnion, and chorion are delivered after the fetus.

Alar plate Dorsal portion of the neural tube.

Allantois Endodermal diverticulum of the yolk sac.

Amnion The innermost membrane surrounding the embryo or fetus. It also forms the epithelial covering of the umbilical cord.

Amniotic fluid Fluid filling the amniotic cavity which cushions the embryo or fetus from external injuries to the mother and allows the fetus to move freely.

Anal membrane A membrane formed from part of the cloacal membrane.

Anal pit The external depression marking the site of the anal membrane. See also *Proctodeum*.

Anencephaly Defective development of the brain and absence of the cranial vault.

Apical ectodermal ridge Thickening of the ectoderm in the distal limb bud tip.

Arm bud Primordium of the arm.

Auricular hillocks Six swellings around the margin of the first branchial groove form the auricle of the ear.

Basal plate Ventral portion of the neural tube.

Bilaminar embryo The early embryo consisting of ectoderm and endoderm layers before the appearance of the mesoderm layer.

Bi-parietal diameter A measurement of the distance between the two parietal bones.

Blastocyst Early embryo consisting of a sphere of trophoblast and embryoblast cells.

Blood islands Hemopoietic (blood-forming) areas on the yolk sac.

Body stalk Stalk connecting the early embryo to the chorion (connecting or umbilical stalk).

Branchial arches Arches in the walls of the neck region and floor of the pharynx.

Branchial grooves Depressions in the ectoderm marking the boundaries of the branchial arches.

Buccopharyngeal membrane The oral membrane which ruptures at about Day 24, linking the mouth and amniotic cavity.

Carnegie Stages A series of developmental stages in early humans devised by R. O'Rahilly and F. Müller.

Caudal Toward the tail, inferior.

Caul An unruptured amniotic sac surrounding the neonate at birth.

Cervical flexure The second brain flexure to appear.

Cervix The neck of the uterus.

Chorion Trophoblast and associated underlying extraembryonic mesoderm.

Chorionic plate The chorion containing the main branches of the umbilical vessels on the fetal placental surface.

Chorionic sac Contains the embryo and its amnion and yolk sac, and is surrounded by the chorion.

Cloaca The dilated terminal part of the hindgut, caudal to the allantoic diverticulum.

Cloacal membrane An area caudal to the primitive streak where the ectoderm and endoderm layers are in contact. Later (Week 6), this membrane is divided to form the anal membrane and the urogenital membrane.

Coelom (intraembryonic) Spaces within the embryo which form the pericardial, pleural, and peritoneal cavities.

Connecting stalk The body or umbilical stalk of the early embryo.

Corona radiata Cells surrounding the ovum after ovulation.

Coronal plane of section A vertical section through the embryo or fetus perpendicular to the median plane.

Cotyledon A unit of the placenta.

Cranial Toward the head, superior, cephalic.

Crown–heel length A straight line measuring the standing height of an older embryo or fetus.

Crown–rump length A straight line measuring the sitting height of an embryo or fetus.

Decidua The endometrium of pregnancy.

Decidua basalis The layer of endometrium underlying the implanted embryo.

Decidua capsularis The layer of endometrium overlying the implanted embryo.

Decidua parietalis All the decidua, other than the decidua basalis and capsularis.

Dental lamina Precursor of the enamel organ.

Dermomyotome Division of the somite which forms the dermis of the skin and skeletal muscle.

Diencephalon Part of the forebrain forming the epithalamus, thalamus, and hypothalamus.

Differentiation Specialization of a cell or a group of cells.

Dorsal Relating to the back.

Ductus arteriosus A blood vessel connecting the left pulmonary artery and aortic arch.

Ductus venosus A blood vessel connecting the left umbilical vein to the inferior vena cava.

Ectoderm The germ layer which forms the nervous system and skin epidermis.

Embryo The fertilized ovum until the end of Week 8.

Embryonic disc The early embryo composed of two or three germ layers before the formation of the body folds.

Enamel organ Precursor of the tooth enamel.

Endoderm The germ layer which forms the gut and its derivatives.

Endometrium Inner layer of the uterus.

Extraembryonic coelom The area outside the embryo which becomes the chorionic cavity.

Extraembryonic mesoderm Mesoderm outside the embryo forming the connective tissue of the chorion, vessels of the umbilical cord and placenta.

Fertilization age The age of the embryo or fetus based on the true date of fertilization of the ovum by the sperm (see *True age*). The gestation period is 38 weeks.

Fetal membranes The amnion, chorion, allantois, and yolk sac remnant.

Fetus The embryo from the beginning of Week 9 to birth.

Flexion The embryo bends to become 'C'-shaped.

Foregut The gut extending from the oral membrane to the point of entry of the common bile duct.

Forewaters In the first stage of labor, amniotic fluid in front of the head escapes when the amnion and chorion rupture.

Genital tubercle The early phallus.

Germ layers The three layers from which all body tissues develop: the ectoderm, mesoderm, and endoderm.

Gravid Pregnant.

Gubernaculum Fibrous tissue attached to the lower end of the gonad, and in the male it is concerned in the descent of the testis.

Hand plate (paddle) The hand primordium.

Head fold Fold in the embryonic disc which forms the head region.

Heart bulge Bulge in the thoracic region over the heart.

Hepatic diverticulum Primordium of the liver and biliary tract.

Hindgut Gut from the distal part of the transverse colon to the superior part of the anal canal.

Horizon A series of developmental stages in early humans devised by G.L. Streeter.

Hyoid arch The second branchial arch.

Implantation The fertilized ovum embedding in the maternal endometrium.

Intraembryonic mesoderm Mesoderm within the embryo.

Labioscrotal swelling Two folds which form the scrotum in the male or labia majora in the female.

Lacuna A small space.

Lanugo The first fine body hair, primarily shed before birth.

Leg bud Primordium of the leg.

Lens placode Precursor of the lens.

Liquor amnii Amniotic fluid.

Longitudinal plane of section A vertical section of the embryo or fetus through the median plane or parallel to it (sagittal).

Mandibular arch The first branchial arch.

Mandibular prominence (process) Part of the first branchial arch which forms the mandible.

Maxillary prominence (process) Part of the first branchial arch which forms the maxilla, zygomatic bone, and squamous temporal bone.

Meconium Green-colored intestinal contents of the late fetus and neonate.

Medial Toward the midline.

Median plane of section A vertical section through the middle of the embryo or fetus, touching both the dorsal and ventral surfaces.

Menstrual age The true age (fertilization age) plus 2 weeks. The gestation period is 40 weeks.

Mesencephalon The midbrain.

Mesoderm The germ layer which forms muscles, connective tissue, and several other tissues within the embryo (see *Extraembryonic mesoderm*).

Mesonephric duct Duct of the mesonephroi, which forms the male ductus deferens.

Mesonephroi Temporary kidney which is replaced by the metanephric kidney.

Metanephric cap Mesoderm cells which collect around the ureteric bud and form the nephrons.

Metanephroi The permanent kidney.

Metencephalon Part of the hindbrain which forms the pons and cerebellum.

Midbrain flexure First brain flexure.

Midgut Gut from the entry of the common bile duct to the distal part of the transverse colon.

Miscarriage An interruption of pregnancy before term (see *Abortion*).

Morula A solid sphere of embryonic cells prior to blastocyst formation.

Multigravida A pregnant woman who has had a previous pregnancy.

Myelencephalon Part of the hindbrain which forms the medulla oblongata.

Neural crest A group of cells dorsal to the neural tube which form most of the peripheral nervous system, pigment cells, meninges, and several other tissues.

Neural folds Two folds which fuse to form the neural tube.

Neural tube Precursor of the central nervous system.

Neuropore Openings at each end of the neural tube, which close later in development.

Notochord An axial cord in the embryo around which organs are laid down.

Oocyte Female germ cell.

Oral membrane See *Buccopharyngeal membrane*.

Otic placode Precursor of the otocyst.

Otocyst Precursor of the inner ear.

Paramesonephric duct Duct beside the mesonephroi. Forms the uterus and uterine tubes.

Paraxial mesoderm Mesoderm which segments into blocks or somites.

Parturition Childbirth, labor.

Phallus Precursor of the clitoris or penis.

Pharyngeal pouches Depressions in the pharyngeal endoderm marking the boundaries of the branchial arches.

Placenta The organ between the fetus and mother for gaseous and metabolic exchange.

Placenta previa A placenta implanted near the internal opening of the cervix which partially or completely covers the cervical opening.

Preaxial border The border of the limb anterior to the axis of the limb.

Polar bodies Minute cells extruded during meiotic division of the oocyte.

Pontine flexure Third brain flexure to appear.

Postaxial border The border of the limb posterior to the axis of the limb.

Primigravida A woman in the first pregnancy.

Primary palate Median palatal process.

Primitive knot (node) An enlargement of the anterior end of the primitive streak.

Primitive streak A thickening of the ectoderm in the trilaminar embryo marking the future position of the notochord and body axis.

Primordial germ cell Precursor of the oocyte or sperm.

Primordium The earliest stage of a structure or organ.

Proctodeum Anal pit or depression.

Pronephroi Early kidney rudiment.

Prosencephalon Forebrain.

Pupillary membrane Mesoderm anterior to the developing lens whose center normally degenerates before birth.

Quickening The fetal movements detected by the mother at 16–20 weeks of pregnancy.

Radial ridges Mesodermal precursors of the fingers and toes.

Rathke's pouch Outpocketing of the stomodeum which forms the anterior and middle lobes of the pituitary.

Rhombencephalon Diamond-shaped hindbrain.

Rostral The relationship of structures to the nose.

Sagittal plane of section A vertical section through the embryo or fetus parallel to the median plane.

Sclerotome Part of the somite contributing to the vertebral column.

Secondary palate Formed from the fusion of the two lateral palatine processes.

Septum transversum Mesodermal partition contributing to the diaphragm.

Sinus venosus Area of blood vessels where the vitelline, umbilical, and cardinal veins converge.

Sperm Male germ cell.

Somatopleure Somatic mesoderm and its related overlying ectoderm.

Somites Segmented blocks of paraxial mesoderm.

Spina bifida A defect of the vertebral arches through which the spinal cord and its membranes may or may not protrude.

Splanchnopleure Splanchnic mesoderm and its related underlying endoderm.

Stomodeum An ectoderm-lined depression at the site of the primitive mouth.

Sulcus limitans Groove separating the alar and basal plates.

Tail fold The caudal body fold marking the caudal end of the embryo.

Telencephalon The two cerebral vesicles.

Thorax Chest.

Transverse plane of section An horizontal section through the embryo or fetus.

Trimester The 9 calendar months of gestation are divided into 3-month periods called trimesters.

Trophoblast The cell layer of the blastocyst which erodes the maternal uterine mucosa and contributes to the placenta.

True age Age from the date of fertilization. Gestation is 38 weeks.

True knot A knot in the umbilical cord.

Truncus arteriosus Region of outflow of the early heart connected to the aortic sac.

Tuberculum impar Median tongue bud.

Ultrasound High frequency sound vibrations passed through tissues to determine and present as a visual display the location and size of areas within the body.

Umbilical cord Cord connecting the fetus and placenta.

Umbilical stalk Stalk connecting the early embryo to the chorion (body stalk or connecting stalk).

Umbilicus Site of the umbilical cord on the body wall.

Urogenital folds External swellings on both margins of the cloacal membrane which form the urethral groove in the male and labia minora in the female.

Urogenital membrane A membrane formed from part of the cloacal membrane.

Urogenital sinus A subdivision of the cloaca.

Urorectal septum Septum dividing the cloaca into the urogenital sinus and rectum and anal canal.

Uterus Womb.

Ventral Relating to the abdomen.

Vertex presentation The crown of the head presenting first in childbirth.

Vernix caseosa Fatty secretion of sebaceous matter and desquamated cells which coats the skin of the fetus.

Wharton's jelly The matrix of the umbilical cord.

Yolk sac A sac enclosed by endoderm in the early embryo.

Zona pellucida Layer between the ovum and corona radiata.

Zygote The oocyte fertilized by a sperm.

Suggestions for Further Reading

Arey, L.B. (1974) *Developmental Anatomy: A Textbook and Laboratory Manual of Embryology.* Revised 7th edition. Philadelphia, W.B. Saunders.

Boyd, J.D. & Hamilton, W.J. (1970) *The Human Placenta.* Cambridge, W. Heffer & Sons.

Crelin, E.S. (1973) *Functional Anatomy of the Newborn.* New Haven, Yale University Press.

Drews, U. (1995) *Color Atlas of Embryology.* Stuttgart, Georg Thieme Verlag.

England, M.A. (1989) *Picture Tests in Embryology.* London, Wolfe Medical Publications.

FitzGerald, M.J.T. & FitzGerald, M. (1994) *Human Embryology.* London, Bailliere Tindall.

Hamilton, W.J., Boyd, J.D. & Mossman, H.W. (1972) *Human Embryology.* 4th edition. Basingstoke, Macmillan Press.

Hinrichsen, K.V. (1990): *Human embryologie. Lehrbuch und Atlas der vorgeburtlichen Entwicklung des Menschen.* Berlin, Springer.

Jirasek, J.E. (1983) *Atlas of Human Prenatal Morphogenesis.* The Hague, Martin Nijhoff.

Larsen, W.J. (1993) *Human Embryology.* London, Churchill Livingstone.

McLachlan, J. (1994) *Medical Embryology.* Wokingham, Addison-Wesley.

Matsumura, G. & England, M.A. (1992) *Embryology Colouring Book.* London, Wolfe.

Moore, K.L. & Persaud, T.V.N. (1993) *The Developing Human: Clinically Oriented Embryology.* 5th edition. Philadelphia, W.B. Saunders.

Nishimura, H. (1983) *Atlas of Human Prenatal Histology.* Tokyo, Igaku-Shoin.

O'Rahilly, R. & Müller, F. (1987) *Developmental Stages in Human Embryos.* Carnegie Institution of Washington Publication 637.

O'Rahilly, R. & Müller, F. (1992) *Human Embryology and Teratology.* New York, Wiley-Liss.

Patten, B.M. (1976) *Human Embryology.* Re-edition. Maidenhead, McGraw Hill.

Sadler, T.W. (1995) *Langman's Medical Embryology.* 7th edition. London, Williams and Wilkins.

Williams, P.L. (1995) *Gray's Anatomy.* 38th edition. London, Churchill Livingstone.

Index